Practical Management of
Skin Cancer

Practical Management of Skin Cancer

Ronald L. Moy, M.D.
Associate Clinical Professor
Division of Dermatology
University of California at
Los Angeles
Los Angeles, California

Daniel P. Taheri, M.D.
Clinical Instructor of Dermatology
Division of Dermatology
University of California at
Los Angeles Medical Center
Beverly Hills, California

Ariel Ostad, M.D.
Clinical Instructor
Department of Dermatology
New York University
School of Medicine
Albert Einstein College of Medicine
New York, New York

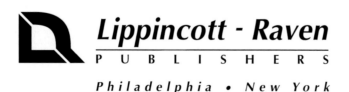

Lippincott - Raven
P U B L I S H E R S

Philadelphia • New York

Acquisitions Editor: Beth Barry
Developmental Editor: Ellen DiFrancesco
Manufacturing Manager: Dennis Teston
Production Manager: Cassie Moore
Production Editor: Kimberly Monroe
Cover Designer: Laura DuPrey
Indexer: Maria Coughlin
Compositor: Maryland Composition

Printed and bound in China.

9 8 7 6 5 4 3 2 1

Library of Congress Cataloging-in-Publication Data

Practical management of skin cancer/editors, Ronald L. Moy, Daniel
   Taheri, Ariel Ostad.
         p.   cm.
   Includes bibliographical references and index.
   ISBN 0-397-51604-5
   1. Skin—Cancer.   I. Moy, Ronald L.   II. Taheri, Daniel.
III. Ostad, Ariel.
   [DNLM: 1. Skin Neoplasms—therapy.   2. Skin Neoplasms—diagnosis.
WR 500P895   1998]
RC280.S5P73   1998
616.99'477—dc21
DNLM/DLC
for Library of Congress   98-30093
                                                                              CIP

*To my wife, Lisa, my daughters, Lauren and Erin,
and my parents, Havard and Jenny.*

Ronald L. Moy

*To my parents, Parviz and Mehry,
and my brother, Michael, for all their love and support.*

Daniel P. Taheri

To my parents for all their love and support.

Ariel Ostad

Contents

Preface

The goal of this textbook is to better familiarize our colleagues in diverse fields of medicine with the various means of diagnosis and treatment of skin cancer. Due to the epidemic rise in the incidence of skin cancer, physicians in all fields of medicine, especially general practitioners, are likely to encounter skin cancer in their practice. Currently, more than 600,000 basal cell carcinomas and 100,000 squamous cell carcinomas are diagnosed yearly in the United States alone. Meanwhile, the incidence of melanoma, the most lethal form of skin cancer, is rising at a rate faster than any other human malignancy.

In *Practical Management of Skin Cancer,* we set out to describe a basic set of guidelines for the appropriate diagnosis and treatment of skin cancer. A variety of skin cancers are described, with particular emphasis on the more common forms of premalignant and malignant skin cancers, including actinic keratosis, Bowen disease, basal cell carcinoma, squamous cell carcinoma, and melanoma and its subtypes.

Diagnostic modalities described include shave biopsy and punch biopsy, as well as the multitude of treatment modalities, including micrographic surgery. Surgical anatomy, proper use of surgical instruments, proper suturing techniques, appropriate postoperative wound care, common surgical complications, and hazardous pitfalls are detailed.

By writing this book, it is our aim to allow our colleagues who do not specialize in the field, particularly those involved in primary care, to obtain a better understanding of skin cancer and, thereby, to allow for its early detection and treatment.

Ronald L. Moy, M.D.
Daniel P. Taheri, M.D.
Ariel Ostad, M.D.

Practical Management of
Skin Cancer

CHAPTER 1

BIOPSY TECHNIQUES

Clinicopathologic correlation is the cornerstone of diagnostic excellence. If used appropriately, the various biopsy techniques can be an important asset to the physician's ability to arrive at the correct diagnosis.

Shave Biopsy

The shave biopsy is an extremely useful way to obtain tissue for diagnostic purposes and for the removal of benign surface neoplasms. It is especially useful for lesions that are somewhat raised above the skin surface and when a full-thickness tissue specimen is not necessary. The shave biopsy is valuable for diagnosing many cutaneous malignancies, including basal cell carcinomas and squamous cell carcinomas. It may also be used in the removal of benign lesions such as seborrheic keratosis and benign melanocytic nevi.

On obtaining informed consent, the site to be sampled is cleansed with an alcohol pad or another antiseptic. The area is then anesthetized by injection of 1% lidocaine with epinephrine.

A 30-gauge needle is inserted into the dermis to raise a wheal. The anesthetic is then injected slowly until blanching of the tissue is seen. On obtaining adequate anesthesia, a no. 15 scalpel blade is held parallel to the skin surface and moved with a straight motion. Simultaneously, the thumb and forefinger of the nondominant hand are used to provide gentle countertraction and stabilize the tissue. In certain anatomic areas, it may be necessary to pinch up the lesion while performing the biopsy. When the tissue has been removed, the biopsy site is blotted with a dry cotton-tipped applicator or gauze to remove any pooled blood. A cotton-tipped applicator dipped in aluminum chloride (Drysol; Person and Covey, Inc., Glendale, CA) is then rolled back and forth over the site. Sometimes, significant pressure needs to be applied with the applicator to achieve hemostasis. Alternatively, ferric sulfate (Monsel's solution) may be used as the hemostatic solution. This has a small risk of causing a "tattooing" of the area, but it is slightly more effective. On achieving adequate hemostasis, a small amount of antibiotic

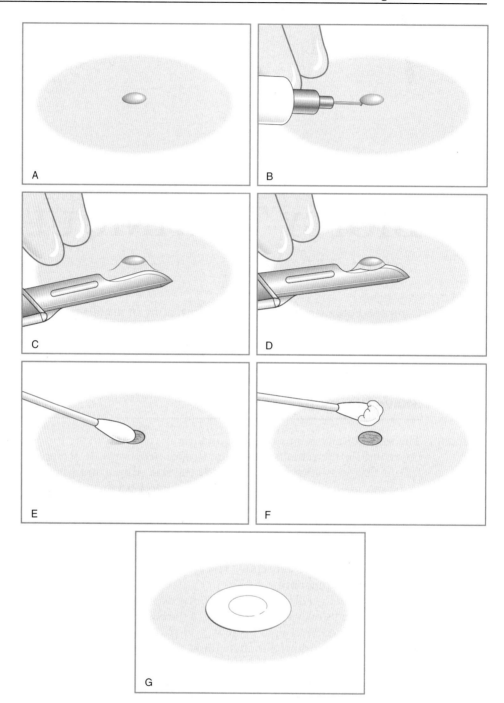

Figure 1

Superficial specimen before injection of anesthetic **(A)**. Local anesthetic injected to raise a wheal around the lesion **(B)**. Shave biopsy with the scalpel blade; the fingers of the non-dominant hand may be used to provide traction **(C)**. The lesion is removed **(D)**. Application of hemostatic agent to stop minor bleeding **(E)**. Antibiotic ointment is applied **(F)**. A simple Band-aid is applied **(G)**.

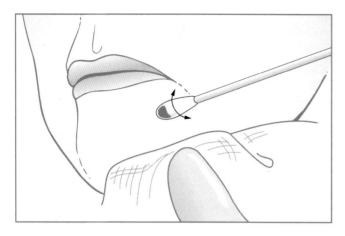

Figure 2
The hemostatic agent is applied to the site using a cotton-tipped applicator, using a rolling, back-and-forth motion.

ointment and a Band-aid are placed over the site. Postoperative instructions for wound care are given to the patient (Figs. 1 and 2; Table 1).

Pigmented lesions and all other lesions suspect for cancer are submitted to the pathologist. If the pathology report indicates that the lesion is benign, no further treatment is necessary. If the report indicates atypical features and the lesion is not

TABLE 1 SHAVE BIOPSY

Indications
  To diagnose
    Actinic keratosis
    Basal cell carcinoma
    Squamous cell carcinoma
    Keratoacanthoma
    Kaposi sarcoma

  To remove
    Seborrheic keratosis
    Benign melanocytic nevi
    Sebaceous hyperplasia
    Pyogenic granuloma
    Skin tag
    Neurofibroma
    Porokeratosis

Contraindications
  Lesion suspect for melanoma

Advantages
  Can be performed rapidly
  Sutures are not needed
  Relatively easy to learn
  An assistant is not needed
  Does not require strict sterile procedure
  Localization of the site after biopsy is not difficult
  Wound care is usually simple
  No restriction of activities needed during the wound-healing period

(continued)

TABLE 1 (Continued)

Disadvantages
  There is an art to mastering the technique
  Hypopigmentation may result
  Scarring may occur over the biopsy site
  A divot may remain if the biopsy is performed too deeply
Equipment needed
  No. 15 blade with scalpel handle
  3-ml syringe with 30-gauge needle
  Cotton-tipped applicators, gauze pads
  Alcohol pad
  Lidocaine with epinephrine
  Specimen bottle with formalin
  Aluminum chloride (Drysol) or ferric sulfate (Monsel's solution)
  Antibiotic ointment
  Band-aid
Complications
  May produce a divot or indentation
  Erythema
  Hypopigmentation
  Regrowth of incompletely excised lesion
  Infection (rare)

completely removed, a complete excision of the lesion may be indicated. If the lesion is indeed malignant, the excision of the entire lesion with appropriate margins of normal tissue must be undertaken. An important note to remember is to avoid the shave biopsy of a lesion suspect for melanoma. This technique does not provide the pathologist with a full-thickness tissue specimen, and therefore the tumor thickness or Clark level cannot be accurately delineated.

Punch Biopsy

The punch biopsy is a procedure that may be used to obtain a full-thickness specimen for histopathologic evaluation (Table 2). It is commonly used to diagnose inflammatory skin conditions for which a full-thickness specimen is needed. It may also be used to assess neoplastic processes such as basal cell carcinoma, squamous cell carcinoma, and melanoma. Punch biopsy is specially advantageous in flat lesions, where the shave technique would leave behind a divot. Because most defects created by a punch biopsy are sutured together, the cosmetic result is usually very good.

If the level of suspicion for melanoma is high, it is preferable to excise the entire lesion to improve the diagnostic yield. If the level of suspicion is low, a punch biopsy may be used to sample the darkest, most elevated, or most suspect area.

Punch biopsy kits come in various sizes, ranging from 2 to 8 mm. A size should be selected that allows for the removal of the lesion with a minimal margin of normal skin. Although reusable steel punches are available, they are rarely used because of the risk of transmission of infectious disease. Disposable punches are easy to use, convenient, and relatively inexpensive.

TABLE 2 PUNCH BIOPSY

Indications
    Diagnosis of
        Inflammatory skin diseases (e.g., lupus, drug eruptions, dermatosis)
        Granulomas—sarcoid, atypical mycobacterial
        Erythema nodosum
        Keratoacanthoma
        Kaposi sarcoma
        Basal cell carcinoma
        Squamous cell carcinoma
        Melanoma
        Cutaneous T-cell lymphoma
    Removal of
        Small nevus
        Neurofibroma

Contraindications
    Caution should be exercised in certain anatomic locations because the procedure can cause damage to deeper underlying structures such as nerves or arteries

Equipment needed
    Punch instrument (2–8 mm)
    Pick-ups
    Fine, curved iris scissors
    Needle driver
    Suture material or hemostatic solution
    3-ml syringe with 30-gauge needle
    Cotton-tipped applicators, gauze pads
    Alcohol pad
    Lidocaine with epinephrine
    Specimen bottle with formalin
    Aluminum chloride (Drysol) or ferric sulfate (Monsel's solution)
    Antibiotic ointment
    Band-aid

Complications
    Induration
    Bleeding (rare)
    Infection (rare)
    Erythema
    Hypertrophic scar
    Excessive protruding skin at edges of scar ("dog-ears")

In contrast to a shave biopsy, a punch biopsy often results in a closed wound, and thus a more rigorous approach to sterile technique is necessary. To perform a punch biopsy, the area is infiltrated with local anesthetic in the same manner as described for a shave biopsy. One percent lidocaine with epinephrine is used except on distal fingers or toes. It is important to infiltrate to the full depth of the dermis, and to allow 10 minutes for the anesthetic to infiltrate the tissue before proceeding. This allows for minimal distortion of tissue while enhancing hemostasis by attaining maximum vasoconstriction.

The punch biopsy instrument should then be placed between the thumb and forefinger and pressed downward with a back-and-forth turning motion. Simultaneously, the nondominant hand should be used to hold tension perpendicular to the relaxed skin tension lines. This tension should be maintained until the dermis is completely separated from the surrounding tissue.

The punch should penetrate completely through the dermis, exposing the subcutaneous fat. Unless in a contraindicated anatomic location, the punch should be driven to the restricted portion of the handle. Stretching the tissue under tension allows the resultant wound, circular under tension, to revert to an oval or fusiform shape. The oval defect will then be aligned with the relaxed skin tension lines, which facilitates closure and optimizes cosmesis (Figs. 3–6).

After penetration of the full thickness of the dermis by the punch instrument, Adsen forceps are used to elevate the specimen, taking care not to crush the tissue. Sharp, curved iris scissors are then used to snip the tissue from the underlying subcutaneous fat. The specimen may then be placed in a 10% buffered neutral formalin container and submitted for pathologic evaluation.

The defect created by the punch may be left to heal by secondary intention (especially for 2-mm punch defects in nonfacial areas), or may be sutured for more rapid and comfortable healing.

Some physicians prefer to use a small amount of Gelfoam placed in the defect to aid in hemostasis. Allowing the punch defect to heal by secondary intention has

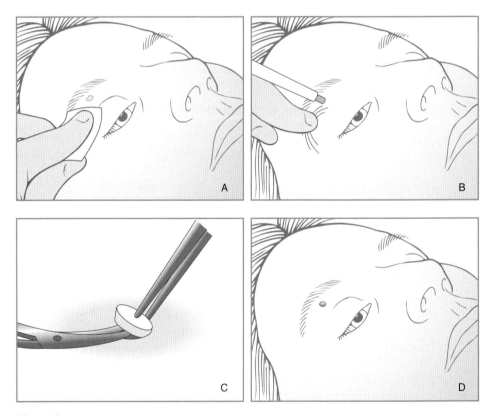

Figure 3

Punch biopsy. After obtaining adequate local anesthesia, an alcohol pad is used to clean the area **(A)**. A punch biopsy instrument is used to create the incision **(B)**. The tissue is gently lifted with forceps and scissors are used to cut the attachments at its base **(C)**. The defect after the procedure **(D)**. At this point, a suture may be used to close the defect.

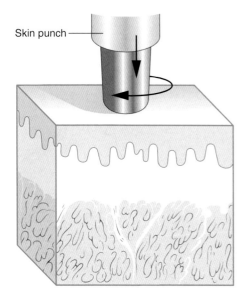

Skin punch

Figure 4
The circular motion applied to the punch biopsy instrument.

its advantages, because it minimizes the risk of needle injury when dealing with patients with hepatitis or acquired immunodeficiency syndrome.

The 3- to 4-mm punch defects are gently closed with one simple stitch, whereas larger punches may require two or more sutures for proper closure (Table 3). Correct suturing technique allows for a better final cosmetic result. The suture placed after a punch is frequently a nonabsorbable suture, such as nylon. There is

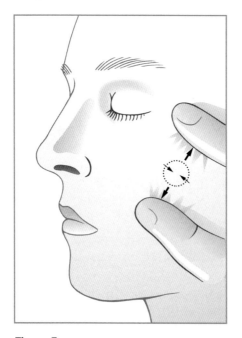
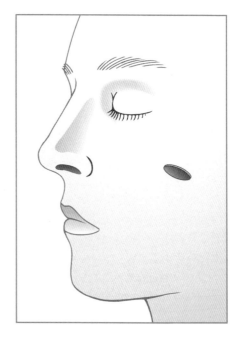

Figure 5
Traction with the fingers of the opposite hand allows for an elliptical defect rather than a circular defect. A better cosmetic outcome is obtained after placement of cuticular stitches.

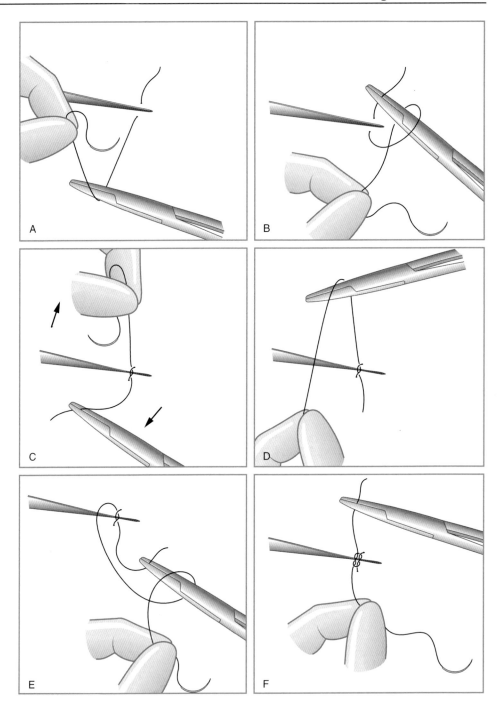

Figure 6

Instrument knot **(A)**. Suture looped over the needle holder **(B)**. Free end of suture grasped with needle holder and pulled through the loop **(C)**. Knot placed to approximate skin edges **(D)**. A second instrument throw in the opposite direction **(E)**. A second knot placed in the opposite direction to the previous one **(F)**. In general, four knots are placed for every suture.

TABLE 3 PUNCH DEFECT CLOSURE GUIDELINES ACCORDING TO SIZE

Size (mm)	Closure
2	Secondary intention or single stitch
3–4	Single stitch
5–8	Two or more stitches

almost never a need for subcutaneous sutures after a punch biopsy. Sutures are usually left in place for 5 to 7 days on the face and 7 to 14 days elsewhere on the body.

Patients should be advised that the resultant scar of a punch biopsy performed in a mobile area such as the arm or the back may stretch with the flexion and extension of muscles. This is especially common in physically active people. In addition, there is the possibility of hypertrophic or keloid scarring in patients with a genetic predisposition.

Compared with elliptical excision, the punch biopsy is an easier and more convenient way to obtain a full-thickness tissue specimen. Complications are extremely infrequent, but an informed consent explaining the risks associated with the procedure should be obtained. These would include the risks of infection, bleeding, and scarring.

Now that we have described the two most commonly used biopsy techniques, we would like to stress the importance of proper documentation. Whenever a biopsy is performed, a procedure note should be written and included in the patient's chart. The procedure note need not be lengthy; in fact, it should be brief and to the point. It is also a good habit to take a Polaroid picture of any lesion suspect for skin cancer before biopsy and to keep it with the patient's chart. Many times, because of inadequate documentation in the patient's chart and good tissue healing after the biopsy, the physician cannot locate the tumor precisely at follow-up. Taking a photograph of the tumor before biopsy and labeling it with a marker pen prevents the treatment of the wrong lesion and may save many headaches! Many successful malpractice cases have arisen from the inadvertent treatment of the wrong spot.

Excisional Surgery

Excisional surgery is the cornerstone of cutaneous surgery. Appropriate preoperative evaluation, proper planning of the procedure, and an understanding of the superficial anatomy is important to achieve a good outcome. This is especially true when performing an excisional surgery on the anatomic structures of the face. A review of facial anatomy is provided in Figures 7 through 12. With experience and attention to detail, the procedure becomes easier to perform and allows for an outstanding cosmetic outcome.

The preoperative evaluation should include screening for bleeding tendencies, the use of aspirin or aspirin-containing products, nonsteroidal antiinflammatory drugs (e.g., ibuprofen), and anticoagulants (Table 4). Other screening questions should include the use of alcohol or tobacco, presence of any allergies to medica-

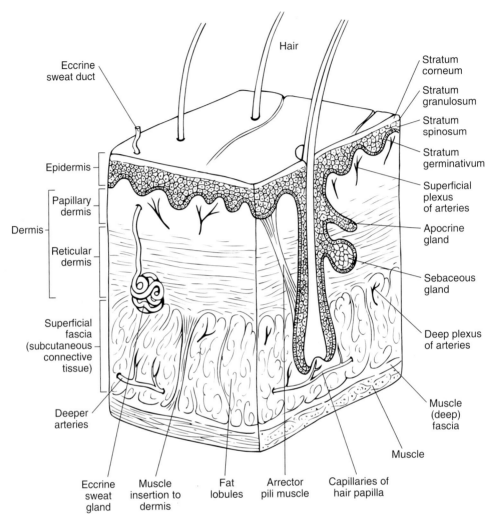

Figure 7

Structure of the skin of the face.

tions, infection with the hepatitis or human immunodeficiency virus, and any tendencies toward abnormal wound healing. At the time of surgery, the lesion is identified and mapped with consideration given to pertinent anatomic structures. Before proceeding, it is a good habit to hand the patient a mirror to ensure that you and the patient agree on the precise location of the tumor. Although it may be hard to believe, many malpractice cases have arisen from treatments performed on the wrong lesion.

In designing the procedure, the first step is to design the excision in the shape of an ellipse.

The next step is to orient the elliptical excision along the natural wrinkle lines of the skin to avoid a conspicuous scar (Fig. 13). If no wrinkles are present, the relaxed skin tension lines should be used to orient the axis of excision.

Another important factor to consider is whether the closure can be accomplished with a side-to-side technique (simple closure). The surgeon can make this

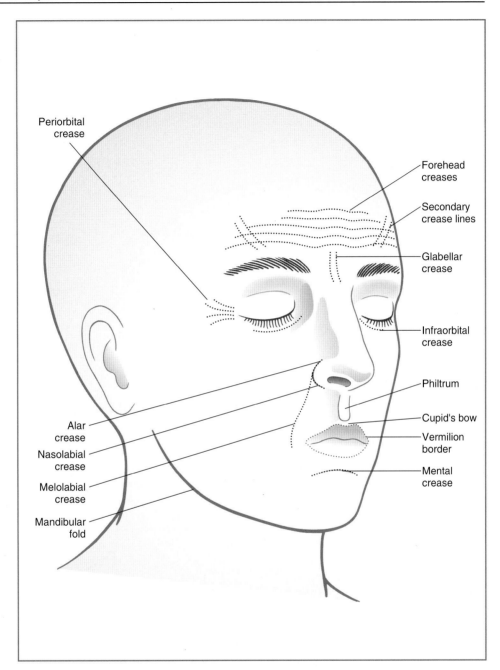

Figure 8
Major landmarks of the face.

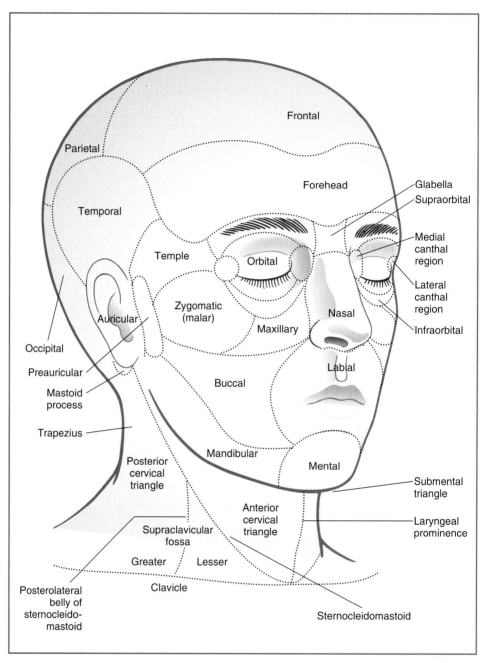

Figure 9

Anatomic regions of the face.

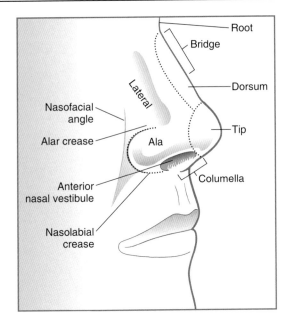

Figure 10
Anatomic regions of the nose.

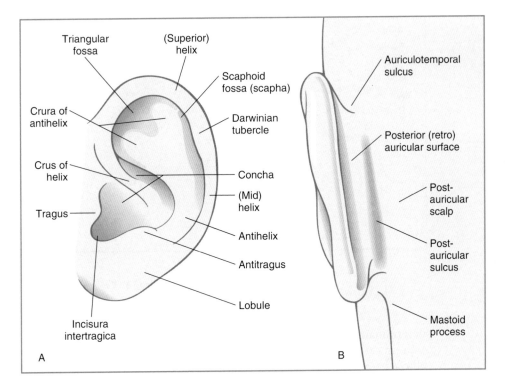

Figure 11
Anatomic regions of the the ear.

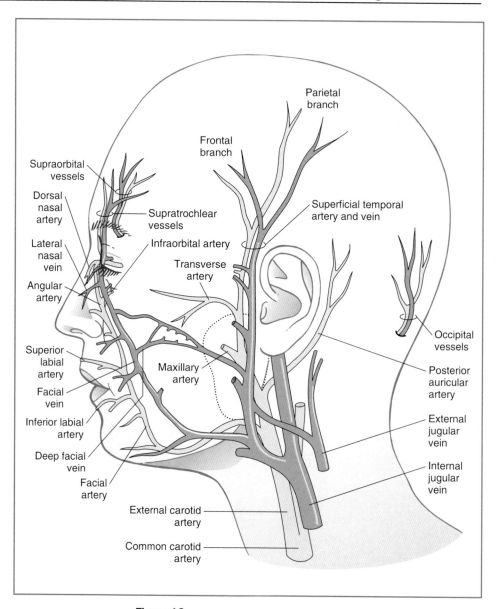

Figure 12
Arterial and venous distribution of the face.

determination by pinching the skin to evaluate the looseness of the skin in the area. In certain anatomic locations, such as near the eyebrow, eyelid, or the lip, the ellipse is oriented so that any pull is in a vertical direction. Any pull in a horizontal direction may result in anatomic distortion.

After cleansing the site with an antiseptic solution, an ellipse is drawn with a surgical marking pen (Jensen Violet pen), following the guidelines outlined previously. The ellipse should usually be designed such that its length is three times its width. It is usually a good idea to make the ellipse longer to avoid the protrusion of tissue, rather than attempt to obtain a shorter scar line. To minimize the

TABLE 4 MEDICATIONS TO AVOID 2 WEEKS BEFORE SURGERY: INSTRUCTIONS TO PATIENT

Advil	Children's aspirin	Feldene	Phenaphen
Alcohol	Clinoril	Fiorinol	Quagesic
Alka Seltzer	Congesprin	4-Way Cold Tabs	Robasisal
Anacin	Cope	Ibuprofen	Rufin
Anaprox	Coricidin	Indocin	Sine-Off
Anaproxin	Coumadin	Indomethacin	Sine Aid
APC	Darvon	Meclomen	Trandate
Ascriptin	Dristan	Motrin	Trental
Aspirin	Easprin	Nalfon	Trilisate
Bufferin	Ecotrin	Naprosyn	Vanquish
Brufen	Empirin	Norgesic	Voltaren
Cephalgesic	Emprazil	Nuprin	Zactrin
Aleve	Cheracol Capsules	Exedrin	Zorpin
			Percodan

If you need minor pain medication, please take acetaminophen (Tylenol) or another nonaspirin medication. Tylenol or Anacin-3 are available at your local pharmacy without a prescription and have comparable pain relief potential to that of aspirin. If you are allergic to acetaminophen (Tylenol) or are unable to take it for other reasons, please notify us so that we can arrange for a suitable substitute.

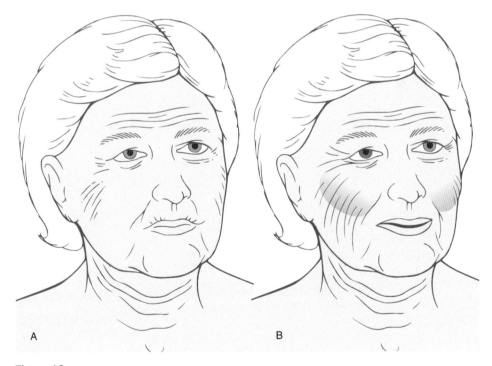

Figure 13

Natural wrinkle lines of the face. The incision should be oriented along these natural lines of the skin.

occurrence of "dog-ears," the ends of the ellipse are excised at approximately a 30-degree angle.

At this time, local anesthesia is obtained using lidocaine with epinephrine. After obtaining adequate anesthesia, the area is resterilized with an antiseptic solution. It is best to wait at least 10 minutes before making the incision. This allows the epinephrine to take effect and thus minimize any bleeding. Conforming to sterile procedure, a scalpel handle holding a no. 15 blade is used for the incision. The scalpel handle should be held perpendicular to the skin and moved with a

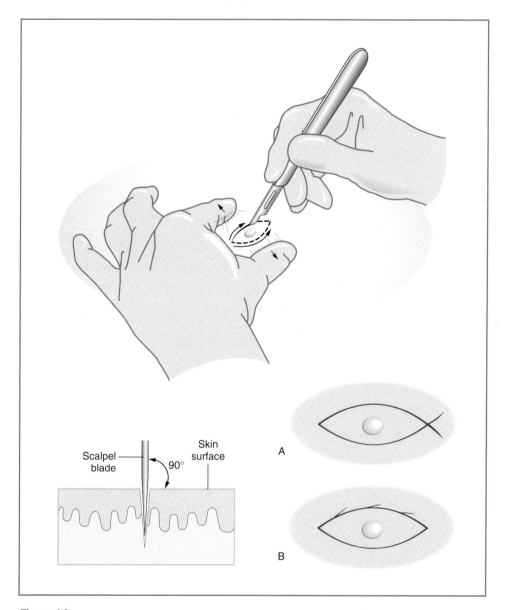

Figure 14

Surgical excision. Scalpel blade should be oriented perpendicular (90 degrees) to the skin surface. Traction should be provided with the opposite hand. Care must be taken to avoid unnecessary incisions that will lead to an undesirable cosmetic outcome. **A:** Do not overcut or go past the end of the incision. **B:** One continuous incision is made pulling toward the surgeon.

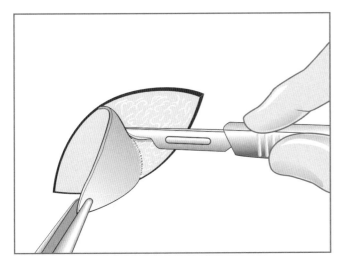

Figure 15

Tissue should be pulled away while cutting the tissue with scalpel blade or suture scissors.

smooth, continuous stroke to allow for a better alignment of the opposite margins (Figs. 14–16). Only the belly of the blade should be used in making the incision, with the tip of the blade used only for the corners of the ellipse. If the scalpel is held at an angle to the skin surface, it will be difficult to obtain a fine-line closure. The depth of the incision should be carried to the underlying subcutaneous fat. Elevating the tissue with forceps at one end, a scalpel or tissue scissors is then used to separate the specimen from the underlying subcutaneous fat. Hemostasis should then be obtained with electrocoagulation as necessary. Although it is important to obtain adequate hemostasis to prevent postoperative bleeding or underlying hematoma formation, it is also important to avoid excess electrocoagulation, because this results in charred, nonviable tissue that may interfere with the proper healing of the wound (Fig. 17).

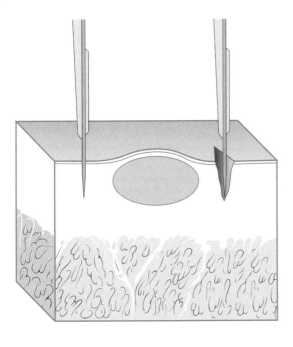

Figure 16

The incision should usually be carried with one pass. Multiple cuts cause a cosmetically unpleasing outcome.

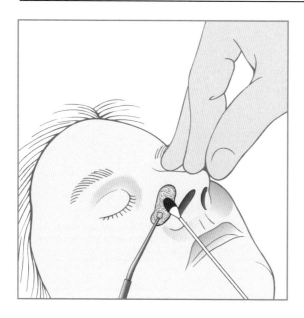

Figure 17
Bleeding may be controlled by applying electrosurgical current to the site. A cotton-tipped applicator may be used to provide a dry field before application of electrosurgical current.

"Undermining," a technique used to decrease tension on the wound edges, may be performed at this time. Here, a surgical blade or tenotomy scissors is used carefully to free the dermis from the underlying subcutaneous fat (Fig. 18). Although most areas of the body are best undermined at the junction of the dermis and the subcutaneous fat, some areas, such as the scalp, are better undermined in a deeper plane, termed the subgaleal space. Undermining should be carried out as extensively as possible to approximate the wound edges without significant tension (see Fig. 18).

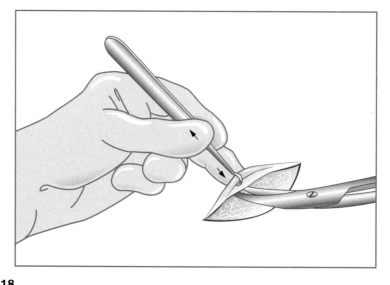

Figure 18
Before placement of sutures, tissue should be undermined. Tissue scissors should be inserted as depicted to allow for greater skin laxity.

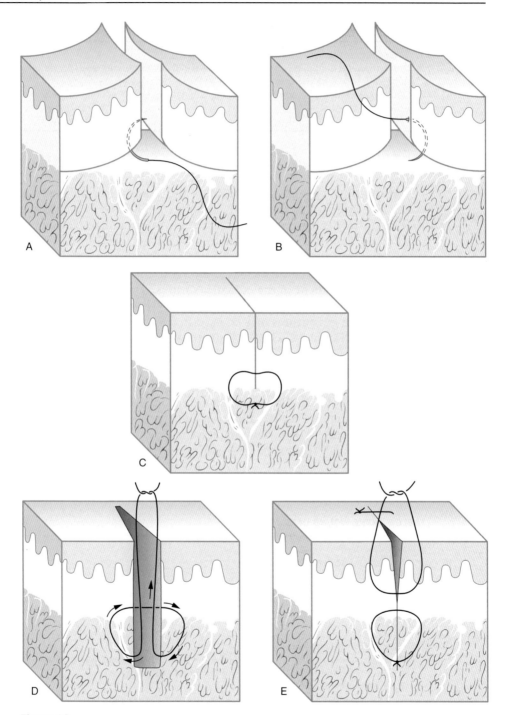

Figure 19

Buried interrupted cutaneous suture. For excisional surgery carried to the level of subcutaneous fat, a buried absorbable suture should be placed, as depicted here. The cuticular suture may then be placed to obtain the final result.

TABLE 5 POSTOPERATIVE WOUND CARE

1. Wound site is cleansed with hydrogen peroxide.
2. Steri-strip tape is applied directly over the wound; adhesive may used for better adhesion.
3. Gauze pad formed into pressure dressing is placed over the wound and held in place with paper tape.

At this time, closure of the defect is undertaken. For the best cosmetic outcome, two layers of suture usually are placed. The first is a subcuticular suture that serves to decrease tension across the wound and to close any underlying dead space. Absorbable sutures such as Dexon or Vicryl should be used for this purpose. A 5-0 subcuticular Dexon or Vicryl suture is usually used for facial defects, whereas a 4-0 subcuticular suture is used for defects on the body. The next step is placement of the cuticular sutures. These primarily serve to attain a better approximation of the wound edges. Nonabsorbable nylon sutures or fast-absorbing gut sutures may be used for this purpose; 6-0 sutures are usually used for facial defects, whereas 5-0 sutures are used for defects on the body (Fig. 19).

After placement of the subcuticular sutures, the surgeon may decide to perform a dog-ear repair. This involves the repair of an elevated cone of tissue at either end of the defect. This can easily be accomplished by extending the incision through the center of the elevated cone of tissue and removing the excess skin using a no. 15 blade. When trimming, it is important to be conservative so as not to remove too much tissue from the end of the ellipse. Finally, it is recommended

TABLE 6 HOME WOUND CARE

Supplies Needed
    Hydrogen peroxide or sterile saline
    Cotton-tipped applicators
    Sterile gauze pads
    Polynmyxin B or bacitracin ointment (not Neosporin)
    Band-aids
Directions
1. Remove the old dressing after 24 hours.
2. Take a cotton-tipped applicator and dip it into hydrogen peroxide or sterile saline. Clean the wound until all serous material and crusts are removed.
3. Apply antibiotic ointment to the wound.
4. Use a Band-aid or a nonstick dressing to cover the wound.
5. The dressing should be changed as above once or twice daily.
6. Tylenol may be taken for pain. The patient should not take aspirin or aspirin-containing products for at least 3 days in after the surgery unless his or her medical history indicates otherwise.

that all dog-ears be excised; otherwise, a cosmetically inelegant bulge of tissue may remain at the edges of the defect.

Before submission of the tissue specimen to the laboratory, the physician should place a suture at one end of the tissue (e.g., the inferior end), and be sure to document this on the patient's chart. If the pathology report reveals residual tumor at a skin edge, the physician may then proceed with a reexcision at that particular margin or refer the patient for Mohs micrographic surgery.

Postoperative Wound Care

After closure, the wound should be cleansed with hydrogen peroxide to remove all debris and blood. Steri-strip tapes are then applied directly over the wound to assist further in the approximation of the skin edges. A gauze pad is then used as a pressure dressing and taped over the wound. Patients are instructed to keep the wound dry for 24 hours. At that time, the pressure dressing is removed but the wound closure tapes are left intact. Antibiotic ointment (polymyxin B or bacitracin) may be applied on top of the wound closure tapes with a new dressing. Wound closure tapes should be left in place until the follow-up visit (Tables 5 and 6). At that time, the sutures are removed and another layer of wound closure tape is applied (Figs. 20–22).

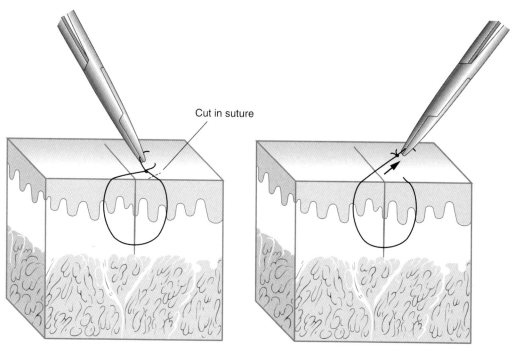

Cut in suture

Figure 20
Suture removal.

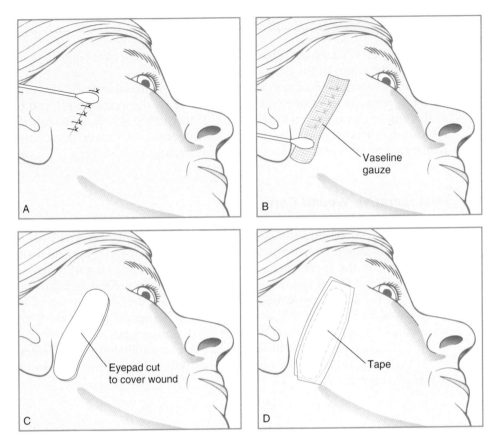

Figure 21

After placement of sutures **(A)**, antibiotic ointment is applied to the wound **(B)**. Gauze and tape may then be used to provide the outer dressing **(C, D)**.

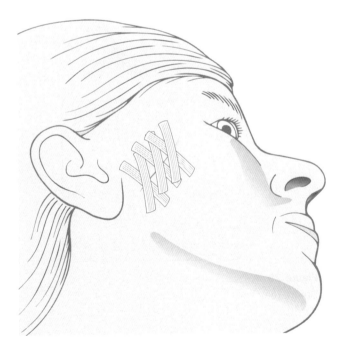

Figure 22

After suture removal, the wound edges may be reinforced with skin closure tapes (Steri-strips).

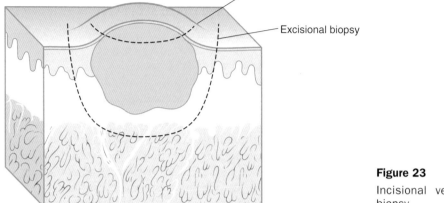

Incisional biopsy

Excisional biopsy

Figure 23
Incisional versus excisional biopsy.

Incisional versus Excisional Biopsy

In the biopsy of any lesion suspect for a nonmelanoma skin cancer, removal of a small portion of the tumor extending into the mid-dermis usually suffices. In general, biopsy and pathologic documentation of skin cancer should be performed *before* proceeding with the excisional surgery of the tumor, because even the most astute clinician can make the wrong clinical diagnosis. Therefore, the biopsies of all nonmelanoma skin cancers are "incisional" rather than "excisional" (only a portion of the tumor is removed at time of biopsy; Fig. 23).

Choosing a particular method of biopsy in treating a pigmented lesion is somewhat more difficult. In contrast to nonmelanoma skin cancers, excisional biopsy (removal of the entire lesion) is the biopsy method of choice. The ability to evaluate the entire surgical specimen under the microscope gives the pathologist a greater opportunity to differentiate a melanoma from a benign entity. This is the reason why a shave biopsy should not be performed on any lesion suspect for melanoma. If a lesion is small enough that it can be removed without significant cosmetic or functional disability, the physician should proceed with the excisional biopsy of the lesion. The biopsy should include 2-mm margins of normal skin. It is a good idea to use a surgical marking pen to draw the incision lines because the anesthesia can cause a distortion of the margins. Another important point to remember is to orient the incision along the path of lymphatic drainage. The depth of the excision should always extend into the subcutaneous tissue, regardless of the nature of the biopsy (incisional or excisional). For larger lesions (>2 cm), an excisional biopsy may not be feasible and an incisional biopsy should be performed. Here, the darkest and most nodular area of the lesion should be selected for biopsy.

Suturing

Suture Selection

In suturing a wound, it should first be realized that there are many different types of sutures available. The lower the number of the sutures needed, the higher the

TABLE 7 CHOOSING SIZE OF ABSORBABLE SUTURES ACCORDING TO TYPE OR LOCATION OF WOUND

Wound	Suture
Wound under tension	3-0 or 4-0
Small wound, not under tension	5-0
Face	5-0

strength and thickness of the suture thread. In general, absorbable subcuticular sutures (buried sutures) are used to remove tension across the wound, whereas nonabsorbable cuticular sutures are used to closely approximate the skin edges.

Subcuticular sutures are important for obtaining wound eversion, providing wound tensile support, and closing dead space (Table 7). Absorbable sutures, in general, lose most of their tensile strength within 60 days after being placed below the skin surface. The type of suture selected depends on the cost and the personal preference of the physician. The most commonly used absorbable sutures are Vicryl and Dexon. With regard to size, the general rule is to use the smallest suture size that will allow for the proper closure of the wound. This reduces the risk of suture tracks and tissue necrosis.

Suturing Technique

Proper suturing technique is essential in achieving good cosmetic results (Table 8). Techniques that must be mastered include eversion of tissue and the precise approximation of skin edges. The natural tendency of sutured wound edges is to become inverted after wound contraction has occurred. By everting the wound edges, a flat rather than an indented scar can be achieved. Wound eversion may be accomplished by everting the wound edges as the needle enters and exits the skin at a 90-degree angle. Furthermore, the path of the needle should be wider at the deepest part of the wound, mimicking a flask (Fig. 24).

When tying the suture, a crucial point to remember is to approximate the skin edges such that they are merely touching each other. If the suture is tied too tightly, it can cause suture marks after postoperative edema, and may even result in tissue necrosis. Knots should be tied and gently pulled to the side of the wound (Fig. 25).

Another important point is the ability of the physician to even out height differences between the wound edges. In general, the needle should enter the skin superficially on the high side and exit the skin deeply on the low side. This allows uneven wound edges to move into the same plane (Fig. 26).

TABLE 8 CORRECT SUTURING TECHNIQUE

1. The suture needle is inserted perpendicular to the skin at the edge of the defect.
2. The needle is then rotated into the opposite site of the wound using a turning wrist motion.
3. An instrument tie is used to tie the suture.
4. Suture should be used to approximate the skin edges.

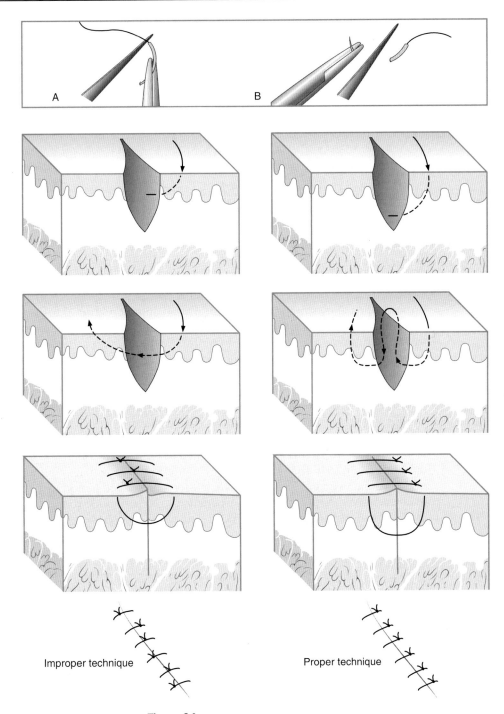

Figure 24
The desired shape is a flask-shaped suture.

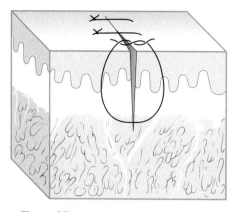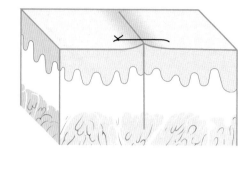

Figure 25

Cutaneous sutures. After tying the knots, they should be pulled to the side of the wound.

There are also many different ways that a suture can be placed, some of which are beyond the scope of the book. The more basic suture is the simple interrupted suture, which allows for a more careful wound approximation. However, it is also more time consuming and more likely to leave railroad-track scars on the skin surface. The running suture is used primarily for wounds that are well approximated and have little tension. The running stitch can be performed quickly and, with experience, can provide the same level of tissue approximation as the simple interrupted suture. However, it is more difficult to master. The vertical mattress suture produces greater wound eversion, closes dead space, and provides increased wound strength across the wound. As the physician gains experience in everting wound edges, this technique is used less often (Table 9).

The outer, nonabsorbable sutures should be removed in a timely fashion to avoid unsightly complications. Sutures that are removed too early may result in dehiscence of the wound, whereas sutures that are left for a prolonged period may result in railroad-track scars. Although clinical experience is the best guide to the appropriate removal of external sutures, some general guidelines are indicated in Table 10.

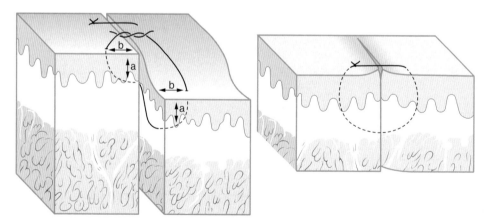

Figure 26

If the epidermal wound edges are uneven, the technique shown here should be used to even them out (high on high side, low on low side).

TABLE 9 SUTURE TECHNIQUES

Simple Interrupted Suture
    Time-consuming technique
    More likely to leave railroad-track scars
    Better able to approximate the skin edges

Running Cuticular Suture
    Can be performed more quickly
    Harder to approximate skin edges
    Tissue dehiscence more likely, especially if not sutured properly

Vertical Mattress Suture
    Produces greater wound eversion
    Closes dead space
    Provides increased wound strength
    More difficulty in closely approximating the wound edges
    May result in prominent suture marks if sutures left in for too long
    Time-consuming technique

Surgical Complications

When a surgical procedure is performed, even under ideal conditions, there is always a risk that complications may develop. It is the role of the physician to recognize any complication early in its course and take the appropriate steps to circumvent it. The most common postoperative complication is scarring. There is a greater risk of scarring when performing surgery on the chest, back, or shoulders, and patients should be appropriately warned of this risk before the procedure is performed. Excessive skin tension or the inappropriate use of sutures can also result in a less appealing scar.

In skin surgery, if good sterile technique is used, the risk of wound infection is relatively low. Because the blood supply is less abundant in the extremities, greater care should be taken when performing surgery in these areas of the body. Redness, warmth, and pain are the classic symptoms of a wound infection.

Excessive bleeding during surgery may occur owing to a multitude of reasons. These include the inappropriate intake of aspirin, nonsteroidal antiinflammatory drugs, and anticoagulants before surgery. Careful hemostasis by electrocoagulation before suturing the wound closed is the key to preventing postoperative bleeding and hematoma formation.

TABLE 10 GUIDELINES FOR REMOVAL OF EXTERNAL SUTURES[a]

Site	Remove After
Face	3–7 days
Neck	5–7 days
Trunk	7–14 days
Extremities	7–14 days
Scalp	7–14 days

[a]Sutures should be left in longer for wounds under greater tension.

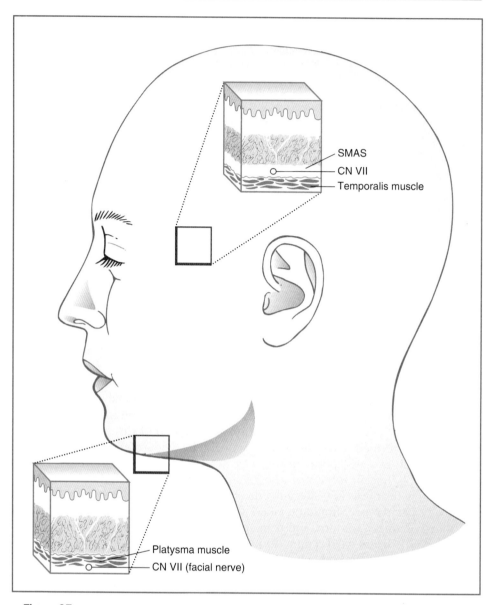

SMAS
CN VII
Temporalis muscle

Platysma muscle
CN VII (facial nerve)

Figure 27

Danger spots: the facial nerve lies especially close to the skin surface in these regions.

Nerve damage is another possible complication of skin cancer surgery. When performing surgery on the head and neck region, the physician should be aware of two nerves that lie fairly superficially in the skin and thus may be damaged during surgery. The first is the temporal branch of the facial nerve, which lies in the superficial subcutaneous fat. This nerve runs between imaginary lines from (1) the tragus to the eyebrow, and (2) the tragus to the upper forehead wrinkle. If this nerve is cut or damaged during surgery, the patient will not be able to wrinkle his or her forehead and may have ptosis (permanent drooping) of the upper eyelid. Damage to the spinal accessory nerve may result in the inability to shrug the shoulder or to initiate abduction of the arm. This nerve also lies fairly superficially, running posterior to the sternocleidomastoid muscle (Figs. 27 and 28).

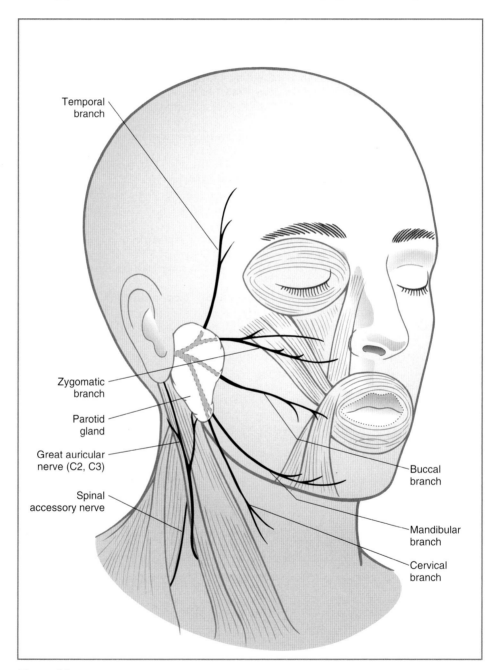

Figure 28

Anatomic locations of the branches of the facial nerve, great auricular nerve, and the spinal accessory nerve.

Suggested Readings

Bart RS, Kopf AW: Techniques of biopsy of cutaneous neoplasms. *Journal of Dermatologic Surgery and Oncology* 1979;5:979–987.

Bennett RG. *Fundamentals of cutaneous surgery.* St. Louis: CV Mosby, 1988.

Bernstein G. Surface landmarks for the identification of key anatomic structures of the face and neck. *Journal of Dermatologic Surgery and Oncology* 1986;12:722–726.

Borges AF. Relaxed skin tension lines versus other skin lines. *Plast Reconstr Surg* 1984;73:144–150.

Chrisman BB. Planning and staffing an appropriate outpatient facility. *Journal of Dermatologic Surgery and Oncology* 1988;14:708–711.

Fitzpatrick TB, Eisen AZ, Wolff K, et al. *Dermatology in general medicine.* New York: McGraw-Hill, 1987.

Larson PO. Topical hemostatic agents for dermatologic surgery. *Journal of Dermatologic Surgery and Oncology* 1988;14:623–632.

Lober CW. Suturing techniques. In: Roenigk RK, Roenigk HH, eds. *Dermatologic surgery.* New York: Marcel Dekker, 1989, pp. 205–217.

Malone B, Maisel R. Anatomy of the facial nerve. *Am J Otolaryngol* 1988;9:494.

Panje WR. Local anesthesia of the face. *Journal of Dermatologic Surgery and Oncology* 1979;5:311–315.

Perry AW, McShane RH. Fine tuning of the skin edges in the closure of surgical wounds. *Journal of Dermatologic Surgery and Oncology* 1981;7:471–476.

Rampen FH, Van der Esch EP. Biopsy and survival of malignant melanoma. *J Am Acad Dermatol* 1985;12:385–388.

Salasche SJ. Acute surgical complications: cause, prevention, and treatment. *J Am Acad Dermatol* 1986;15:1163–1185.

Salasche SJ, Bernstein G, Senkarik M. Surgical anatomy of the skin. Norwalk, CT: Appleton & Lange, 1988.

Stegman SJ. Planning closure of a surgical wound. *Journal of Dermatologic Surgery and Oncology* 1978;4:390–393.

Stegman SJ. Suturing techniques for dermatologic surgery. *Journal of Dermatologic Surgery and Oncology* 1978;4:63–68.

Stock AL, Collins HP, Davidson TM. Anatomy of the superficial temporal artery. *Head Neck Surg* 1980;2:466–469.

CHAPTER 2

SKIN CANCER TREATMENTS

Electrodesiccation and Curettage

Although basal cell carcinoma (Fig. 1) is the most common lesion treated by electrodesiccation and curettage, a variety of superficial skin lesions may be removed using this technique (Table 1). The instruments used in this technique include a set of sharp dermal curettes and an electrodesiccation unit.

In performing this procedure, local anesthesia is first obtained using lidocaine and epinephrine (Fig. 2A). A sharp dermal curette such as a 2-0 or 3-0 is used to scrape out the tumor. To debulk the tumor, the curette is held like a pencil and moved in many different directions (see Fig. 2A,B). Simultaneously, the surrounding skin is spread taut with the nondominant hand. The curette moves through the basal cell carcinoma with relative ease because the tumor is friable. The goal here is to create a uniform char at the base and the sides of the curetted lesion. The charred tissue is then removed with a curette. The cycle of desiccation and curettage is repeated twice. Studies have shown that three cycles of curettage and electrodesiccation as described are more likely to diminish the possibility of recurrence of the tumor. Special care should be taken adequately to treat the edges of the lesion because recurrences of this skin cancer are most likely to arise from this area. After completion of treatment, antibacterial ointment and wound dressing are applied to the area.

When treating a patient with this modality, a few important points should be considered. Alcohol is a flammable material and should not be used to prepare the skin. During treatment, the patient should not grasp or touch the metal portions of the treatment table. It is also a good idea to use a smoke evacuator with the intake nozzle held within 2 cm of the operative field. There is a potential risk of transmission of hepatitis or even human immunodeficiency virus through the smoke plume. Although there is little scientific evidence for such transmission, surgical masks and eye protection should be worn at all times. In patients known

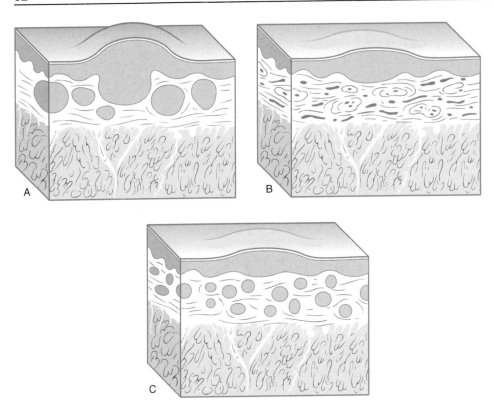

Figure 1
Different patterns of basal cell carcinoma: nodular **(A)**, sclerosing **(B)**, and micronodular **(C)**.

TABLE 1 LESIONS THAT MAY BE TREATED WITH ELECTRODESICCATION AND CURETTAGE

Basal cell carcinoma	
Bowen disease	} Curette, then electrodesiccate. Repeat 2×
Squamous cell carcinoma (low-risk)	

to be infected with a transmissible disease, a different treatment modality may be considered based on the evaluation of risks and benefits of treatment (Tables 2 and 3). Electrosurgery should also be avoided in patients with pacemakers. If there is no alternative, a cardiologist should be consulted to discuss the risks and benefits for the patient based on the type of pacemaker and stability of the patient (Table 4).

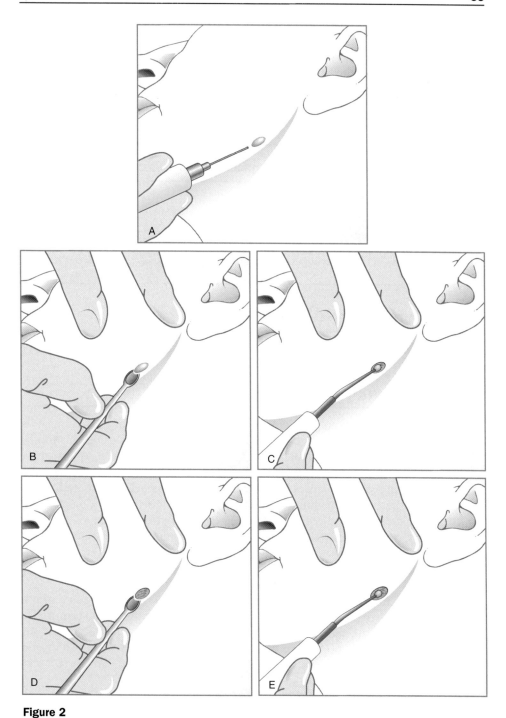

Figure 2

Electrodesiccation and curettage of basal cell carcinoma. After obtaining adequate anesthesia **(A)**, the lesion is curetted **(B)** and then coagulated **(C)**. This is then repeated to ensure complete clearing of the tumor **(D, E)**.

TABLE 2 ADVANTAGES OF ELECTRODESICCATION AND CURETTAGE

Simple to use, easy to master
Rapid technique
Controls bleeding while destroying tissue
Equipment compact and affordable
Sterile procedure not necessary
Wound infection rare

TABLE 3 DISADVANTAGES OF ELECTRODESICCATION AND CURRETAGE

Risk of electric shock
Hypertrophic scar
Smoke may carry viral particles
Unsightly wound
Home wound care required for prolonged period
Margins of tissue cannot be evaluated histologically because of tissue destruction

Surgical Excision

This treatment modality uses the techniques outlined in Chapter 1.

Cryosurgery

Cryosurgery is an excellent modality for the treatment of superficial basal cell carcinoma. However, great care should be exercised in using this modality to treat malignant lesions. Table 5 lists the possible complications of cryotherapy.

The use of a thermocouple (a probe to measure the tissue temperature) when treating skin malignancies with cryotherapy has been advocated.

Before proceeding with treatment, it is important to obtain a definitive pathologic diagnosis. Because of the existence of better techniques and the steep learning curve associated with the use of the thermocouple, we advocate the treatment only of superficial basal cell carcinomas with this technique. Relative contraindications by area are neoplasms of the ala nasi and nasolabial fold, anterior tragus, and the upper lip near the vermilion border.

During treatment, liquid nitrogen is applied with a cryogun to the center of the lesion such that an ice ball starts to form in the center of the tumor. This is continued until the halo extends 5 mm around the tumor. The freeze time should extend approximately 60 to 90 seconds. The halo thaw time should also extend to over 60 seconds. Cure rates of 90% to 95% have been reported with correct technique.

TABLE 4 CONTRAINDICATIONS TO ELECTRODESICCATION AND CURRETAGE

Patient with pacemaker, metal plates, or pins
Melanoma (electrosurgery should never be used to treat any pigmented lesion even remotely suspect for melanoma)
Certain types of basal cell carcinoma (e.g., sclerosing basal cell carcinoma), large tumors, or those located in sensitive locations
Large or aggressive subtypes of squamous cell carcinoma

TABLE 5 COMPLICATIONS OF CRYOSURGERY

Immediate
    Edema
    Headache
    (Blistering and pain in the immediate postoperative period is a regular and expected finding)
Delayed
    Infection
    Hyperpigmentation
    Hypertrophic scar
    Milia
    Neuropathy
Permanent
    Hypopigmentation
    Ectropion
    Tenting of the vermilion border of the upper lip
    Skin atrophy
    Alopecia

The two most common postoperative effects of cryotherapy include pain and blistering. Table 6 is a sample consent form that lists possible risks. The patient should be advised either to allow the blister to resolve spontaneously or to drain it with a sterile needle. If the roof of the blister is opened to the outside, antibiotic ointment and a sterile dressing should be applied.

Intralesional Therapy

A number of experimental protocols have been investigated or are under study for the treatment of skin neoplasms. They are beyond the scope of this book, and are not discussed here any further.

Radiation

Radiation therapy for skin cancers is primarily reserved for those patients who are poor candidates for surgery. It is also used as adjuvant therapy for those patients with deeply invasive or metastatic skin cancer. Radiation therapy is primarily practiced by radiation oncologists. Advances in the field now allow for a significantly lower complication rate compared with the older treatment protocols.

The single most important advance in radiation therapy of tumors is the fractionation of the total dose of radiation over several treatments. This allows for the delivery of a higher total dose with a better tissue response. Various forms of radiation may be used in the treatment of skin cancer, including soft x-rays, electron-beam, and grenz-ray radiation. The specific modality used depends on the specific clinical circumstance. The treatment is usually painless and well tolerated by the patient.

The disadvantages of radiation treatment include its incapacity to provide a pathologic specimen to evaluate the adequacy of treatment, and the necessity for

TABLE 6 SAMPLE CONSENT FORM FOR CRYOSURGERY

The surgical procedure or treatment to be performed is called cryosurgery.
I, _____ hereby consent to the surgical procedure or treatment
that has been explained to me. I understand the following are possible risks involved:

1. Pain
2. Bleeding
3. Infection
4. Scar formation
5. Persistent redness
6. Increase or decrease of my skin pigmentation
7. Recurrence of the skin lesion
8. Paresthesia (local nerve damage or numbness)
9. Fainting

I understand there may be other methods to do this procedure, but agree to the procedure about
to be done, understanding all risks. I have been given the opportunity to ask all my questions
regarding the procedure and its risks. I agree that photographs may be taken.

Patient's signature   Guardian's signature

Date   Date

multiple treatment sessions. The postoperative period is followed by radiation dermatitis, which consists of erosion and exudation of the treated tissue. Depending on the extensiveness of treatment, the healing period may take up to 8 weeks, and requires prolonged wound care. The treated area usually becomes cosmetically compromised, with atrophy and discoloration common findings. Radiation therapy for skin cancers on the trunk or extremities should be discouraged because of delayed healing and poor cosmetic outcome.

Mohs Micrographic Surgery

Mohs micrographic surgery represents a major advance in the treatment of skin cancer (Table 7; Fig. 3). It entails the sequential excision of the skin cancer, using appropriate mapping, frozen sectioning, staining, and microscopic examination of the tissue to ensure the complete removal of the entire base and perimeter of the skin cancer. This procedure is indicated for removal of difficult tumors with indistinct clinical margins. The technique is especially useful for lesions in cosmetically important areas.

The surgery is performed under local anesthesia in an outpatient setting. It does not require overnight hospitalization. Similar to other surgical procedures, appropriate preoperative evaluation must be undertaken. Aspirin should be discontinued for 2 weeks and alcohol for 5 days before the procedure. Lidocaine 1% with 1:200,000 epinephrine is usually used to obtain local anesthesia. For more

TABLE 7 ADVANTAGES OF MOHS SURGERY

Highest cure rate of any treatment modality
Conservation of normal tissue, allowing for a better cosmetic result
Performed under local anesthesia
Outpatient surgery

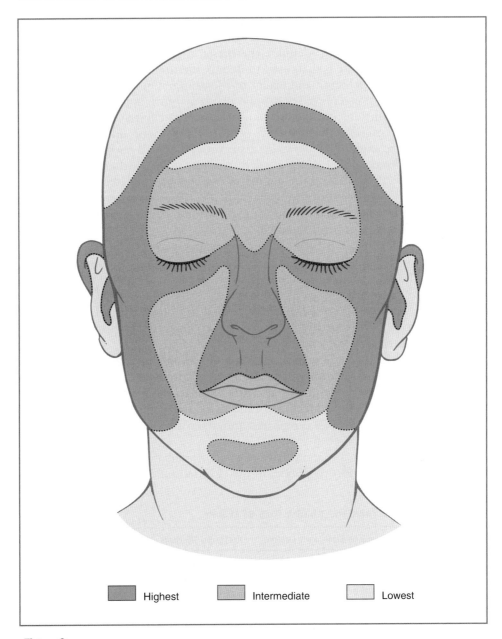

Figure 3

Skin cancer recurrence rates. (From Lambert DR, Siegle RJ. Skin cancer: a review with consideration of treatment options including Moh's micrographic surgery. *Ohio Medicine* 1990;86:745, with permission.)

involved tumors and those located in sensitive locations, local nerve blocks may sometimes be used to obtain regional anesthesia.

On achieving adequate anesthesia, the area is prepared as in a standard excision. A curette is then used to debulk the tumor. Curetting helps better to identify the true depth and extent of the tumor. Using a scalpel with a no. 15 blade, the tumor is removed with appropriate margins (approximately 2 to 3 mm of normal tissue around the tumor) based on the clinical characteristics of the tumor. While excising this first layer of tissue, it is important to bevel the sides at a 45-degree angle. This allows for easier processing and microscopic visualization of the entire cut surface. If the angle of excision is deeper, the tissue cannot be processed correctly and the entire cut margin cannot be evaluated.

On removal of the tissue, superficial incisional nicks are placed through the specimen as well as the surrounding wound margin so that exact orientation of the specimen can be maintained.

The tissue is then stained and mapped to correlate its exact location on the body. The tissue may be divided into two or more sections before being frozen. This is important because it is difficult for larger pieces of tissue to lay flat in a two-dimensional plane.

A cryostat is used to cut horizontal sections of the frozen tissue specimen measuring 6 to 10 μm in thickness. The sections are then placed on a microscope slide and typically stained with hematoxylin and eosin for microscopic evaluation. If any residual tumor is demonstrated, its location is marked accordingly on the map. Any remaining tumor is then removed by excising another thin layer of skin from the area of the wound that corresponds to the marked area on the map. During the processing and reading of the slides, the patient may wait in the waiting room. This whole process is repeated until microscopic evaluation finds all margins clear of tumor.

Once clear margins have been confirmed around the tumor, the surgeon evaluates the defect to decide on the closure modality that would best preserve nor-

TABLE 8 TREATMENT MODALITIES BY LESION

Premalignant or Malignant Lesion	Preferred Method	Alternative Method
Actinic keratoses	Cryosurgery	Electrosurgery
	Topical agents	Shave excision
Keratoacanthoma	ED&C	Cryosurgery
	Elliptical excision	Shave or punch excision
Lentigo maligna	Elliptical excision	
	Cryosurgery	
Melanoma (includes lentigo maligna melanoma)	Excision or Mohs surgery, based on tumor characteristics	
Bowen disease	Elliptical excision	
	Cryosurgery	
	Electrosurgery	
	Shave excision	
Basal cell carcinoma	ED&C, excision or Mohs surgery, depending on tumor characteristics	

ED&C, electrodesiccation and curettage.

TABLE 9 TREATMENT MODALITIES FOR NONMELANOMA SKIN CANCER

Surgical excision: Treatment of choice for nodular basal cell carcinomas and medium-sized
  squamous cell carcinomas
    Advantages
        Optimal cosmetic result when repair is immediate
        Rapid healing
        Margin control
    Disadvantages
        Time consuming
        Technically difficult
        Potential complications: bleeding, hematoma, infection
Electrosurgery: Treatment of choice for small nodular and superficial basal cell carcinomas and
  small squamous cell carcinomas
    Advantages
        Quick procedure
        Technically easy to perform
    Disadvantages
        Prolonged healing period
        No margin control
        Cosmetic result variable
Cryosurgery: Treatment of choice for superficial basal cell carcinomas
    Advantages
        Quick procedure
        Good cosmetic result
    Disadvantages
        Prolonged healing period
        No margin control
Radiation therapy: Treatment of choice for patients who are not operative candidates
    Advantages
        Good cosmetic result
    Disadvantages
        Multiple treatment sessions
        High cost
        Postoperative sequelae such as scarring and long-term carcinogenesis
Mohs surgery: Treatment of choice for sclerosing and recurrent basal cell carcinomas and large
  squamous cell carcinomas
    Advantages
        Best cure rates of any treatment modality
        Meticulous margin control
    Disadvantages
        Time consuming
        Technically difficult
        High cost

mal anatomic and functional relationships and allow for the best cosmetic outcome. Depending on the defect, the tissue may be allowed to heal by granulation
and epithelialization (secondary intention healing), it may be closed primarily, or
it may require a skin flap or a skin graft.

Mohs surgery is more expensive than other treatment modalities already mentioned (Tables 8 and 9). The other methods of tumor destruction remain cost effective in the treatment of primary tumors in areas where the tumors have a tendency not to recur and wide surgical margins would not compromise the cosmetic
results. Table 10 lists the possible postoperative complications of skin surgery.

TABLE 10 POSSIBLE POSTOPERATIVE COMPLICATIONS OF SKIN SURGERY

Within the first 2 weeks
  Infection
  Pain
  Bleeding
  Dehiscence
  Hematoma
  Bruising and swelling
  Suture spitting

Late complications
  Scarring
  Hypertrophic scars
  Keloid
  Hyperpigmentation or hypopigmentation
  Nerve damage
  Ectropion or entropion of eyelids
  Tenting or notching of the vermilion border of the upper lip
  Skin atrophy
  Alopecia
  Recurrence of the lesion

Suggested Readings

Boneschi V, Brambila L, Chiappino G, et al. Intralesional alpha-2B recombinant interferon for basal cell carcinomas. *Int J Dermatol* 1991;30:220–224.

Brady LW, Binnick SA, Fitzpatrick PJ. Skin cancer. In: Perez CA, Brady LW, eds. *Principles and practice of radiation oncology.* Philadelphia: JB Lippincott, 1987, pp. 377–394.

Cooper JS. Radiotherapy in the treatment of skin cancer. In: Friedman RJ, Rigel DS, Kopf AW, et al, eds. *Cancer of the skin.* Philadelphia: WB Saunders, 1991, pp. 553–568.

Gage AA, Kuflik EG. *Cryosurgical treatment of skin cancer.* New York: Igaku-Shoin, 1990, pp. 65–82.

Greenway HT, Cornell RC, Tanner DJ, et al. Treatment of basal cell carcinoma with intralesional interferon. *J Am Acad Dermatol* 1986;15:437–443.

Hunter RD. *Radiotherapy of malignant disease.* New York: Springer-Verlag, 1985, pp. 135–151.

Mohs FE. Mohs micrographic surgery: a historical perspective. *Dermatol Clin* 1989;7:609–611.

Roenigk RK. Mohs micrographic surgery. *Mayo Clin Proc* 1988;63:175–183.

Sebben JE. *Cutaneous electrosurgery.* Chicago: Year Book Medical, 1989.

Spiller WF, Spiller RF. Treatment of basal cell epitheliomaby curettage and electrodesiccation. *J Am Acad Dermatol* 1984;11:808–814.

Stegman SJ, Tromovitch TA. Modern chemosurgery: microscopically controlled excision. *West J Med* 1980;132:7–12.

Torre D. Cryosurgery of premalignant and malignant skin lesions. *Cutis* 1971;11:123–129.

Tromovitch TA. Skin cancer: treatment by curettage and desiccation. *California Medicine* 1965;103:107–108.

Zacarian SA, Adham MI. Cryotherapy of cutaneous malignancy. *Cryobiology* 1966;2:212–218.

CHAPTER 3

Basal Cell Carcinoma

Definition

Basal cell carcinoma (BCC) is a malignant neoplasm of the skin that is composed of cells that resemble the basal cell layer of the epidermis and its appendages (Figs. 1–26). It is believed that the neoplastic cells derive from keratinocyte stem cells located in the basal cell layer of the skin, as well as the germinative cells of hair follicles. BCC is the most common cancer in humans. Over 500,000 cases of BCC are diagnosed in the United States annually. BCC is a slow-growing tumor that rarely metastasizes. The incidence of metastasis is less than 0.1% of all tumors, with almost all cases either due to the "basosquamous" form of the tumor or those occurring in immunocompromised hosts. BCC outnumbers squamous cell carcinoma (SCC) by a factor of approximately four to one.

The incidence of BCC increases greatly with chronic sun exposure (Figs. 27–33). It is more frequent in men than in women, with most cases occurring in white people older than 40 years of age. Eight percent of BCCs arise on the sun-exposed skin of the head and neck, with the nose accounting for approximately 30% of all cases. Despite its indolent nature, BCC can cause extensive local tissue destruction (Figs. 34–58). If not treated early in its course, significant functional and cosmetic impairment may result.

(Text continues on page 65)

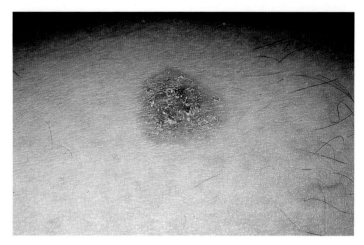

Figure 1
Superficial basal cell carcinoma with erythema and crusting.

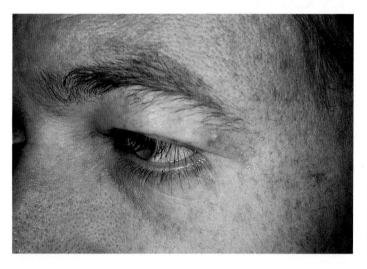

Figure 2
Basal cell carcinoma. This tumor is located in a cosmetically sensitive area, on the lateral aspect of the upper eyelid.

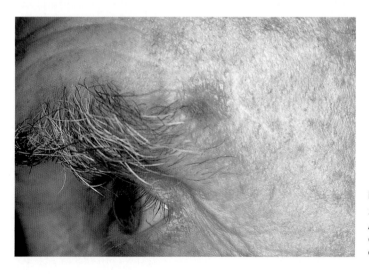

Figure 3
Superficial basal cell carcinoma. A pink patch with pearly borders on the lateral aspect of the upper eyelid.

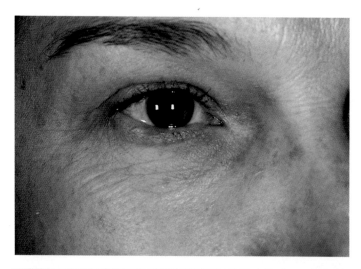

Figure 4

Basal cell carcinoma. This tumor is located on the vermilion border of the lower eyelid.

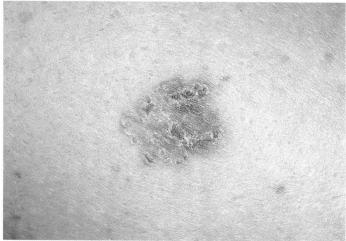

Figure 5

Superficial basal cell carcinoma. A pink, scaling plaque located on the trunk.

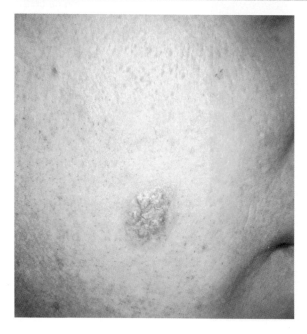

Figure 6

Basal cell carcinoma. Translucent, well circumscribed nodule on the right cheek of a patient in her mid-30s.

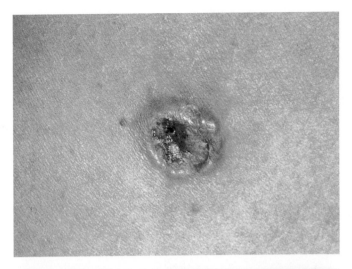

Figure 7

Note the characteristic "pearly" (shiny) borders of this basal cell carcinoma. Central ulceration of the tumor is also seen.

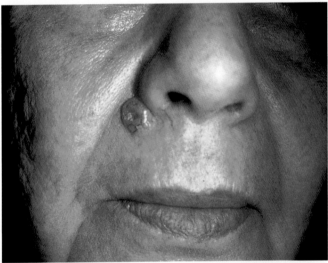

Figure 8

Nodular basal cell carcinoma on the medial aspect of the alar crease.

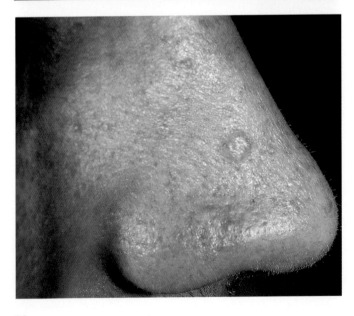

Figure 9

A fairly inconspicuous, flesh-colored basal cell carcinoma on the right side of the nose. A shave biopsy confirmed the diagnosis.

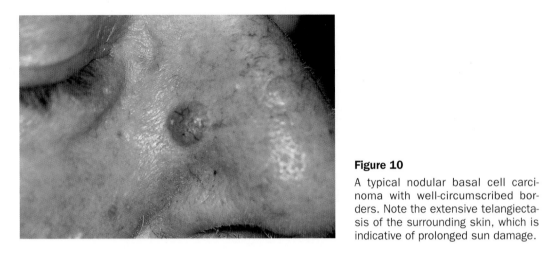

Figure 10

A typical nodular basal cell carcinoma with well-circumscribed borders. Note the extensive telangiectasis of the surrounding skin, which is indicative of prolonged sun damage.

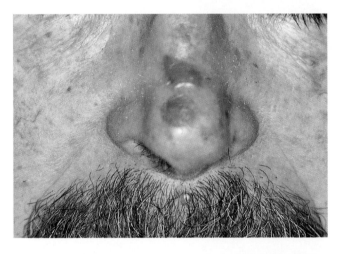

Figure 11

Two basal cell carcinomas located in close proximity on dorsum of the nose. Mohs surgical excision of the tumors revealed tumor in the intervening, normal-appearing skin.

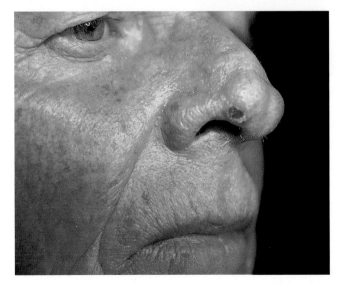

Figure 12

Basal cell carcinoma on the right alar rim in a light-complected man.

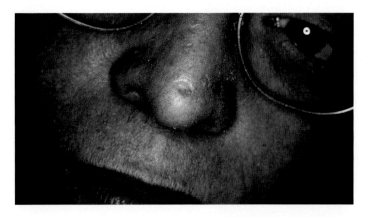

Figure 13
Basal cell carcinoma resembling a scar on the supratip of the nose.

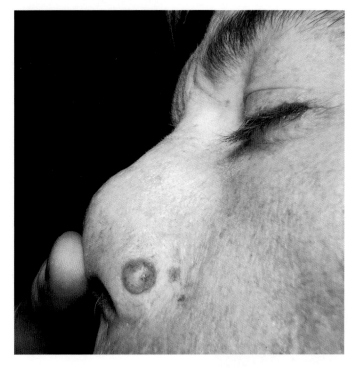

Figure 14
Nodular basal cell carcinoma on the left nasal ala.

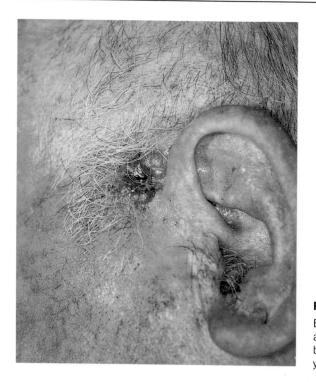

Figure 15

Basal cell carcinoma on the left preauricular area. This patient has had multiple other basal cell carcinomas excised in preceding years.

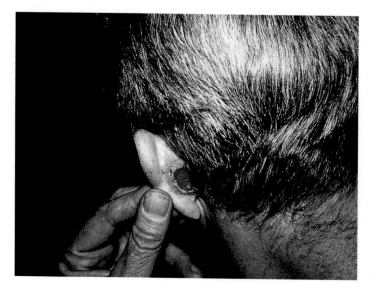

Figure 16

Ulcerated basal cell carcinoma on the posterior aspect of the left ear, emphasizing the necessity for a thorough cutaneous examination.

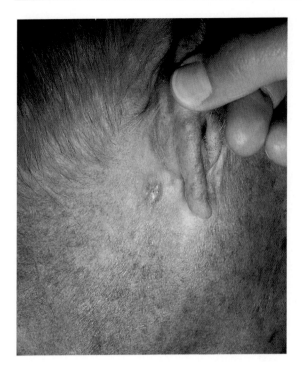

Figure 17

Pearly pink papule on the right postauricular skin. The clinical presentation is characteristic.

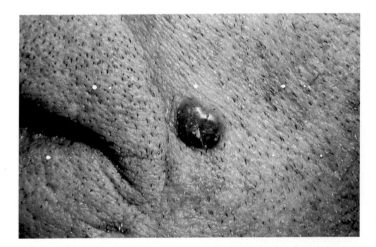

Figure 18

Pigmented basal cell carcinoma bordering the left nasolabial fold. This form of basal cell carcinoma can sometimes mimic malignant melanoma.

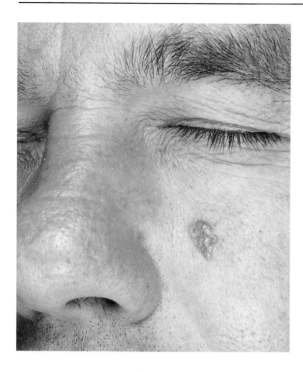

Figure 19

Basal cell carcinoma with poorly delineated borders on the left medial cheek.

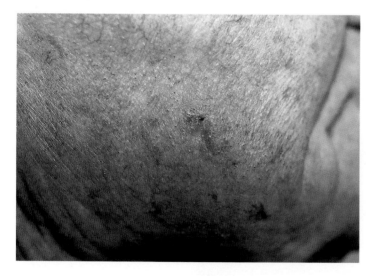

Figure 20

Staged surgical excision of the tumor using the Mohs technique showed extensive subclinical extension of the tumor beyond visible margins.

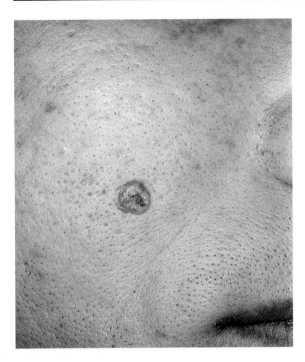

Figure 21
A typical-appearing basal cell carcinoma on
the right cheek.

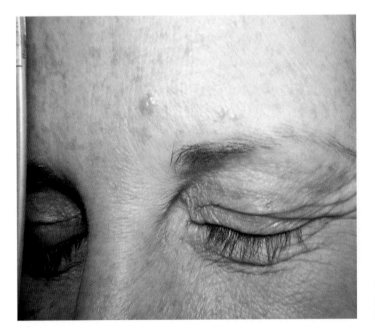

Figure 22
Basal cell carcinoma on the forehead in a middle-aged woman.

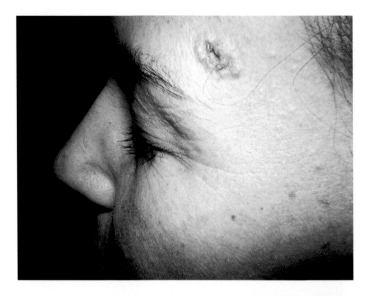

Figure 23

A basal cell carcinoma on the left temple that had been neglected for many months. Excision of this tumor should proceed with caution because the ophthalmic branch of the facial nerve lies in this region.

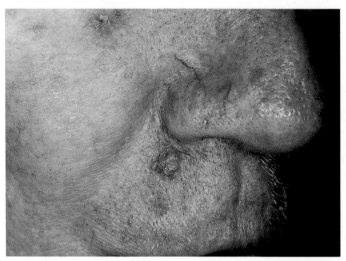

Figure 24

Basal cell carcinoma on the right upper lip.

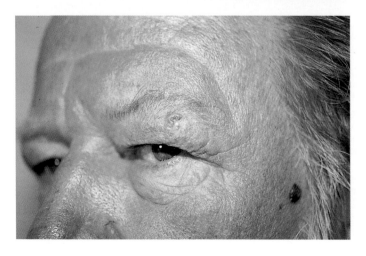

Figure 25

Basal cell carcinoma of the left upper eyelid.

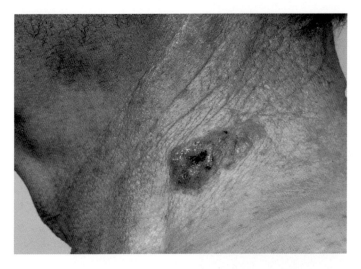

Figure 26
Basal cell carcinoma on the lateral aspect of the neck. This tumor had been neglected for over 1 year.

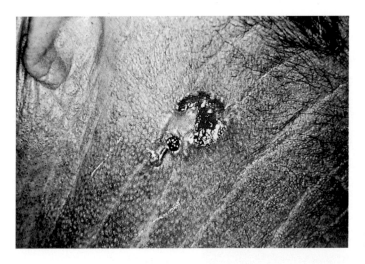

Figure 27
Basal cell carcinoma on the left posterior neck. The deep furrows are indicative of extensive sun damage.

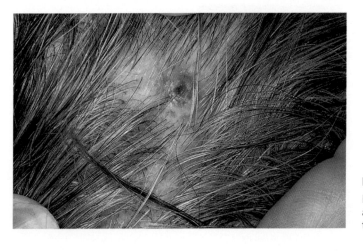

Figure 28
Basal cell carcinoma on the scalp—a somewhat unusual location for this tumor.

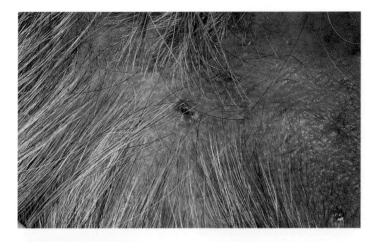

Figure 29

Basal cell carcinoma on the scalp.

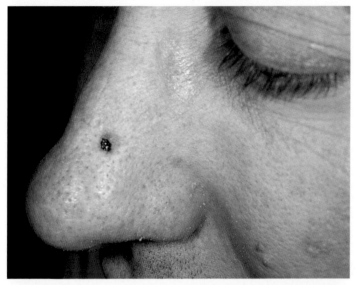

Figure 30

Basal cell carcinoma on the nose in a patient in her late 20s. Tumors are being seen in the younger population with a greater incidence.

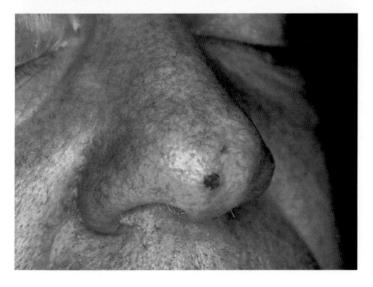

Figure 31

Basal cell carcinoma on the tip of nose. All cutaneous sites may be susceptible.

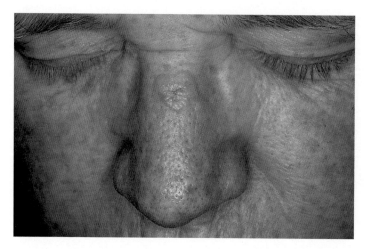

Figure 32

Basal cell carcinoma on the dorsum of nose. Note the freckles and the light complexion. People who sunburn easily are at a significantly greater risk.

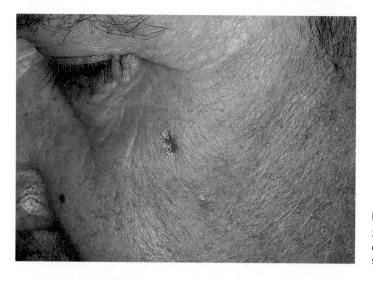

Figure 33

Sclerosing basal cell carcinoma on the right cheekbone. Note the scar-like appearance of the tumor.

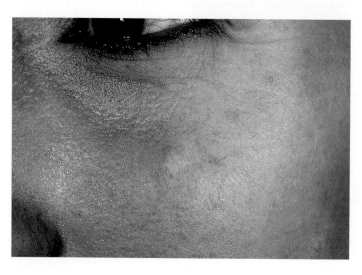

Figure 34

Sclerosing basal cell carcinoma on the left cheek presenting as a white, translucent, atrophic papule. Note that the characteristic features of basal cell carcinoma are missing.

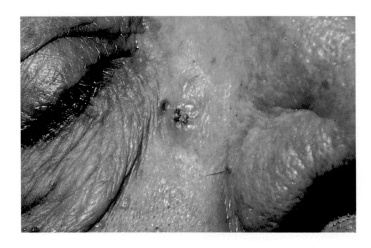

Figure 35
Basal cell carcinoma. Note the poorly defined margins.

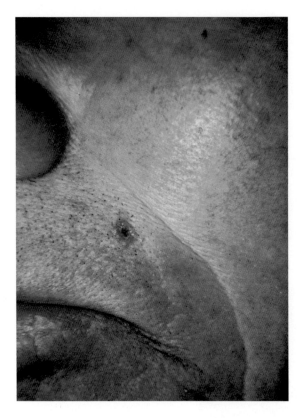

Figure 36
Basal cell carcinoma on the left upper lip.

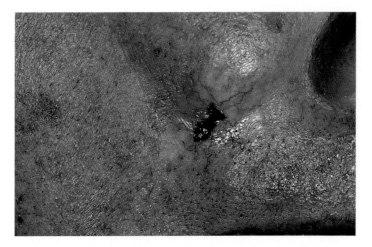

Figure 37

Sclerosing basal cell carcinoma on the right nasolabial fold. This tumor has a high recurrence rate with the traditional therapeutic modalities. Mohs surgery is the gold standard in treating this tumor.

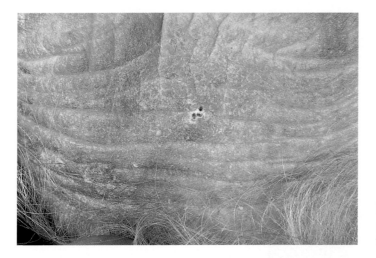

Figure 38

Basal cell carcinoma on the mid-forehead.

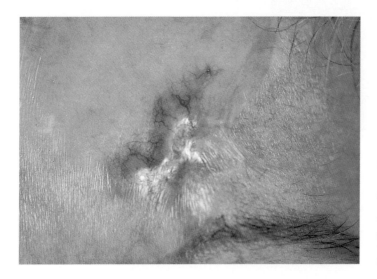

Figure 39

Recurrent sclerosing basal cell carcinoma on the superior aspect of the left eyebrow. This form of basal cell carcinoma had an aggressive growth pattern, frequently invading muscle, nerve, and bone.

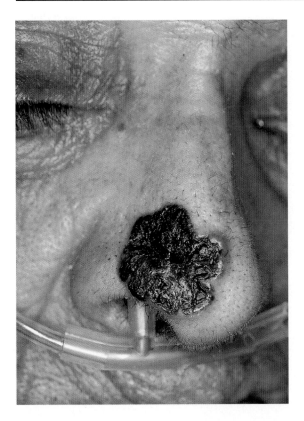

Figure 40

Large pigmented basal cell carcinoma in an elderly white woman with multiple medical problems. Note the well-defined borders and the dark pigmentation.

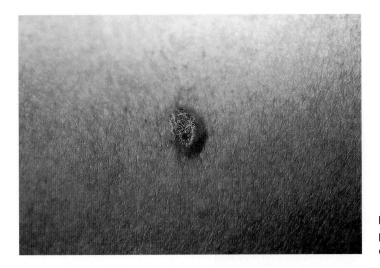

Figure 41

Pigmented basal cell carcinoma on the trunk.

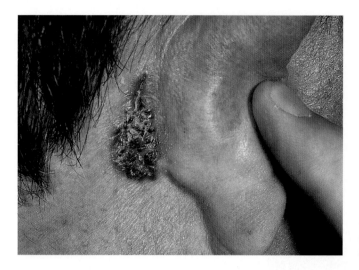

Figure 42
Basal cell carcinoma on the right postauricular skin. The presence of melanin gives the tumor an unusual appearance.

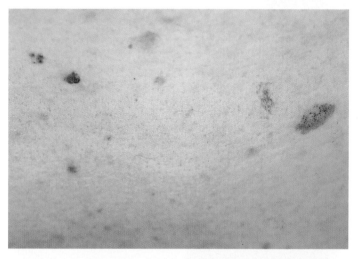

Figure 43
Two pigmented basal cell carcinomas on the left upper side of the photograph. A blue nevus and a seborrheic keratosis are also seen.

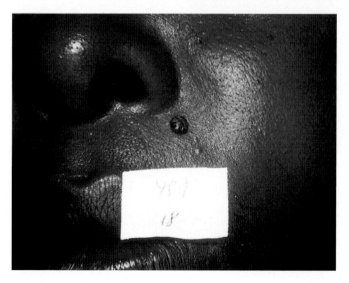

Figure 44
Pigmented basal cell carcinoma in a black patient.

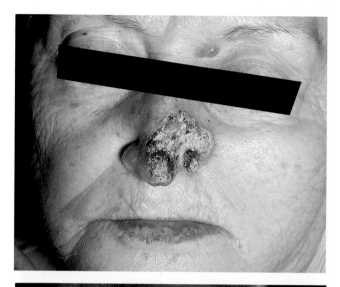

Figure 45

An unusual verrucous basal cell carcinoma that covers a large portion of the nose. This women had tried unsuccessfully to cover the tumor with makeup. A second tumor is present on the left upper eyelid skin.

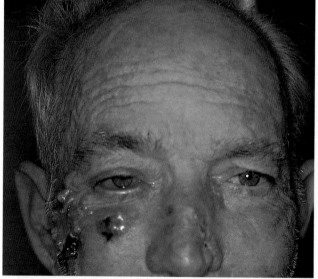

Figure 46

Multiple large basal cell carcinomas in an elderly man.

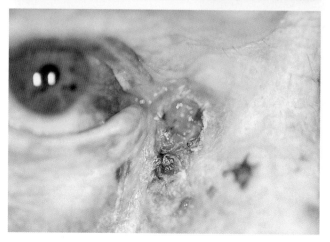

Figure 47

Large basal cell carcinoma near the eye. Note the rolled borders and the ulcerated center. Mohs surgical evaluation of the peripheral and deep margins is a necessity if recurrence is to be avoided.

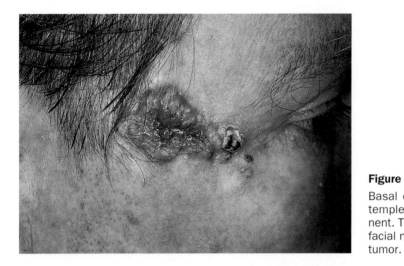

Figure 48

Basal cell carcinoma on the right temple with a pigmented component. The ophthalmic branch of the facial nerve tracks underneath this tumor.

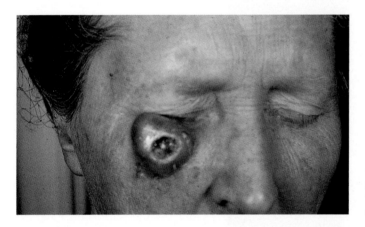

Figure 49

An advanced basal cell carcinoma that has encroached onto the right eye.

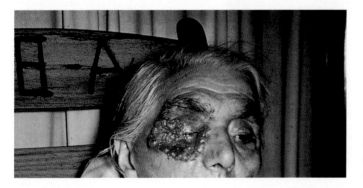

Figure 50

Extensive basal cell carcinoma in an elderly woman.

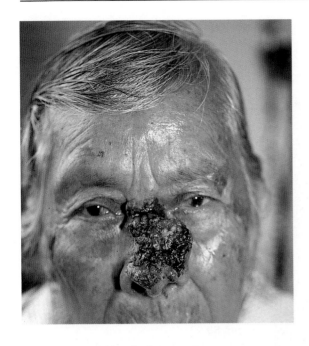

Figure 51

Advanced basal cell carcinoma involving the entire nose. If neglected, the tumor will continue to spread locally. Although rare, metastatic spread can occur.

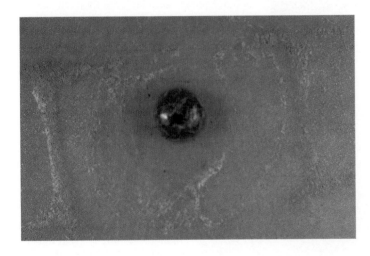

Figure 52

Pyogenic granuloma. This is a benign vascular tumor that may be mistaken for a basal cell carcinoma or a melanoma.

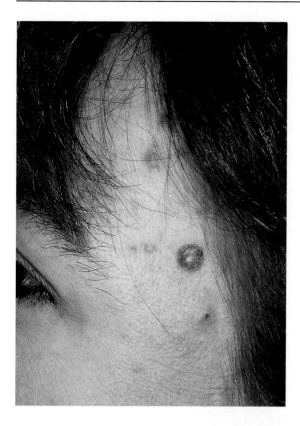

Figure 53

Angiolymphoid hyperplasia with eosinophilia, another benign vascular tumor that tends to occur around the ears. Distinguishing this tumor from a basal cell carcinoma may at times be difficult.

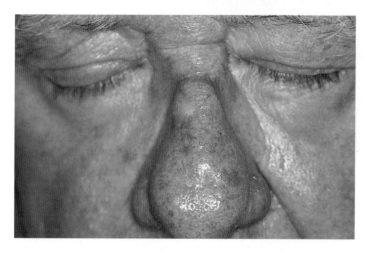

Figure 54

Basosquamous cell carcinoma appearing as a slightly depressed plaque on the nose. Presenting with features of both basal cell and squamous cell carcinoma, this form of the tumor is diagnosed based on its histologic appearance.

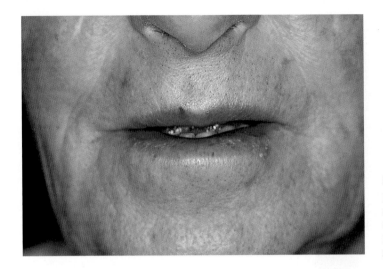

Figure 55

Basosquamous cell carcinoma on the left lower vermilion border of the lip. Involvement of the lip mucosa indicates a more aggressive clinical course.

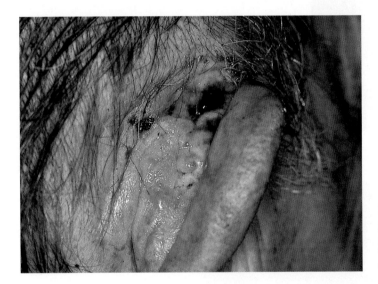

Figure 56

Basosquamous cell carcinoma on the right postauricular skin. This tumor is more aggressive than a basal cell carcinoma.

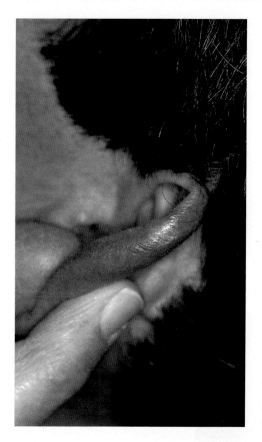

Figure 57
Basosquamous cell carcinoma on the left helical rim.

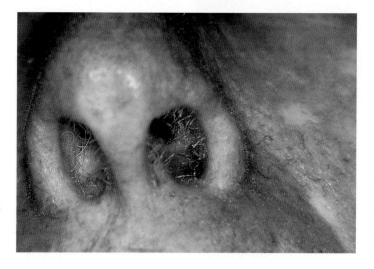

Figure 58
Basosquamous cell carcinoma inside the left nostril. An unusual location, but a reminder that skin cancer can occur on virtually any cutaneous surface.

TABLE 1 RISK FACTORS FOR DEVELOPMENT OF BASAL CELL CARCINOMA

Fair skin, poor tanning ability
Ultraviolet light
Immunosuppression
Genetic predisposition
Ionizing radiation
Arsenic exposure
Congenital hamartoma

Risk Factors

The most common risk factor for the development of BCC is ultraviolet light (Table 1). Heavy sun exposure, outdoor occupations, inability to tan, and Scottish, Scandinavian, or Irish descent are all significant factors in the development of BCC. People with fair complexion who sunburn easily are at a significantly increased risk. The dark-skinned population has a much lower propensity toward development of BCC. Cumulative exposure to ultraviolet light, not periodic bursts of exposure, is most significantly correlated to the development of BCC.

Basal cell carcinoma occurs more frequently and at a younger age in immunosuppressed people. An increased incidence of BCC has been observed in transplant recipients who are on immunosuppressive medication. Similarly, patients who are immunosuppressed because of a variety of other diseases, including lymphoma, leukemia, and acquired immunodeficiency syndrome, are similarly affected. BCC in these patients tends to occur in sun-exposed sites and is significantly more aggressive. Although relatively uncommon, scars arising from trauma, vaccinations, tattoos, and burns may give rise to BCC over time. Other risk factors include exposure to arsenic, either through its past medicinal use or through contaminated water supplies. Arsenic-induced BCCs are usually multiple and mostly occur in sun-protected sites.

Ionizing radiation may also cause the delayed development of BCC. This form of therapy was used in the past in treating a variety of benign skin conditions, including acne, eczema, and tinea capitis.

Genetic diseases also predispose to the development of BCC. In people with so-called "basal cell nevus syndrome," a rare autosomal dominant genetic disorder, multiple BCCs develop at a very early age. In xeroderma pigmentosum, a rare autosomal dominant disorder, patients are extremely sensitive to ultraviolet light and have multiple skin cancers at a very early age.

Pathogenesis

Multiple theories have been proposed to explain the origin of BCC (Table 2). Although the histologic variants of BCC do not correlate with any one particular epithelial structure, BCC is generally considered to arise from epidermal stem cells. Therefore, BCC can differentiate to any epithelial structure. Its clinical behavior is mainly influenced by the adjacent dermis. This "stromal dependence" accounts for the extremely low incidence of metastasis.

TABLE 2 MECHANISMS OF ULTRAVIOLET LIGHT–INDUCED FORMATION OF BASAL CELL CARCINOMA

Keratinocyte DNA mutation
Localized immunosuppression

The most common etiologic factor in the induction of BCC is ultraviolet light. The wavelength most important in the development of BCC is ultraviolet B (UVB; 290–320 nm). Animal studies have shown that sunscreens that block UVB decrease the incidence of skin cancer. Gradual depletion of the ozone layer, which filters out short-wavelength ultraviolet light, has further added to the increased incidence of BCC. Ultraviolet A (UVA; 320–400 nm) readily penetrates the dermis but is less carcinogenic than UVB. However, the combination of the two results in a potent carcinogenic stimulus.

Ultraviolet light mediates carcinogenesis through epidermal DNA damage. It has been shown that ultraviolet light induces characteristic DNA mutations, such as pyrimidine dimers. The *p53* tumor suppressor gene is responsible for arresting the cell cycle such that any induced mutations can be repaired. In BCC, the same ultraviolet light–induced pyrimidine dimer mutations have been found in the *p53* tumor suppressor gene. A mutated and hence nonfunctional *p53* gene leads to dysregulation of the cell cycle, with consequent unlimited cell proliferation. DNA damage also plays a critical role in ionizing radiation-induced BCC.

The role of the immune system in the regulation of BCC is not completely understood. It has been demonstrated that ultraviolet light induces a state of immunosuppression that allows skin cancers to develop and grow. UVB depresses the Langerhans cells, which are responsible for antigen processing and the initiation of the immune cascade in the skin. It also increases the number of T-suppressor cells while decreasing the number of natural killer cells. This leads to a state of immune tolerance, resulting in unsuppressed tumor growth. Advancing age also causes a similar decrease in the number of Langerhans cells. This decrease in immune function is at least partly responsible for the development of BCC in the elderly as well as immunosuppressed people.

Clinical Characteristics

Early lesions of BCC commonly present with a small, translucent papule with a pearly (shiny) raised border containing ectatic blood vessels (Table 3). The tumor is not scaly or hyperkeratotic, but can present with superficial crusting.

Basal cell carcinoma has a variety of distinct clinicopathologic subtypes (Table 4). These include nodular, cystic, adenoid, pigmented, superficial, and morpheaform patterns.

Noduloulcerative or nodular BCC begins as a small, firm, dome-shaped, translucent papule with telangiectases running across the surface. This lesion may periodically erode and eventually ulcerates if left untreated. This form of BCC may spread deeply and cause local tissue destruction.

Superficial BCC appears as a red to pink, scaling plaque with occasional shallow erosions. It occurs more commonly on the trunk and extremities and is seen

TABLE 3 CLINICAL DIFFERENTIAL DIAGNOSIS OF BASAL CELL CARCINOMA

Nodular Type	Superficial Type	Pigmented Type	Sclerosing Type
Sebaceous hyperplasia	Eczema	Melanoma	Scar
Squamous cell carcinoma	Psoriasis	Nevus	
Verruca	Bowen disease		
Molluscum contagiosum			
Intradermal nevus			
Appendegeal tumors			
Amelanotic melanoma			

more commonly in patients with a history of arsenic or radiation exposure. Patients may have multiple small lesions that are disconnected yet cover a large area of the skin, such as the back. These tumors enlarge peripherally and rarely penetrate into the dermis. Superficial BCC may be confused with SCC-*in-situ* (Bowen disease), and a biopsy may be required to differentiate between the two entities.

The morpheaform or sclerosing variant of BCC occurs exclusively on the face. In this form, there is a dense fibrosis of the connective tissue that clinically appears as a characteristic, indurated white plaque with an atrophic surface. This form of BCC has an aggressive growth pattern, frequently invading muscle, nerve, and bone. This tumor can escape notice because of its benign, scar-like appearance. In addition, this type of BCC has indistinct clinical margins with subclinical extensions far beyond the clinically visible borders. Therefore, sclerosing BCC has a high recurrence rate with the traditional treatments used in eradicating the tumor.

TABLE 4 CLINICAL/HISTOLOGIC SUBTYPES OF BASAL CELL CARCINOMA

Noduloulcerative
    Most common type
    Often with overlying telangiectases or ulceration
    Pearly (shiny) border
    Most commonly occurs on the face

Superficial
    Most common on the trunk
    Pink to reddish scaly papule/plaque

Pigmented
    Brown pigmentation
    Mimics melanoma clinically

Morpheaform (sclerosing)
    Flat, indurated white plaque
    Appears as scar
    Smooth, shiny surface
    Indistinct borders
    More aggressive behavior
    Most commonly located on face

Basosquamous
    Has no consistent clinical feature—can occur in any location
    Histologic diagnosis a must
    Aggressive clinical behavior, increased likelihood of metastases

Basosquamous or metatypical BCC is a pathologic entity that is diagnosed on histologic grounds. It has features of both BCC and SCC, and is associated with a higher rate of metastatic spread.

All forms of BCC grow by direct extension and invasion of contiguous structures.

Diagnosis

Clinical recognition of a BCC may be difficult because of its resemblance to other clinical entities. In its initial stages, the nodular pattern of BCC may be mistaken for sebaceous hyperplasia, molluscum contagiosum, or an intradermal nevus. A shave biopsy of the lesion may be needed to confirm the diagnosis. Although not common, scaling and crusting of BCC may occur, causing it to simulate actinic keratosis and SCC.

Some BCC tumors contain pigment and are referred to as "pigmented BCC." The tumor may be confused with melanoma or a seborrheic keratosis. The most difficult problem is encountered in differentiating superficial BCC from isolated patches of eczema, psoriasis, or SCC-*in-situ* (Bowen disease). A shave biopsy is needed to make this diagnosis.

Pathology

Basal cell carcinoma has a very characteristic histologic appearance. The tumor cells are basophilic, and possess only a small amount of cytoplasm with "peripheral palisading." This refers to an orderly line of basal cells along the periphery of tumor nests in the dermis. The proliferation of cells produces a characteristic palisading at the margin, with a cleft separating the tumor from the surrounding stroma.

Treatment

A variety of treatment modalities may be effective in treating BCC (Table 5). It is the physician's responsibility to take the various clinical and histologic parameters into account before deciding on the treatment modality. The factors that should be considered include the location and size of the tumor, whether it is a primary or recurrent tumor, its histologic pattern, and the general health of the patient.

Cryosurgery

Freezing with liquid nitrogen has been advocated for the treatment of superficial forms of BCC as well as the smaller tumors of the nodular type (Table 6). It is not indicated for tumors deeper than 3 mm or those with indistinct margins.

TABLE 5 RECOMMENDED TREATMENT OF BASAL CELL CARCINOMA DEPENDING ON TYPE

Type	Treatment
Noduloulcerative	
<1 cm on face (except the T-zone and folds): primary lesion	ED&C Surgical excision
<1 cm on face (T-zone): periorbital, ears, nose, lip, and nasolabial folds	Mohs micrographic surgery
>1 cm on face — any location	Mohs micrographic surgery
Any size lesion on trunk or extremities	ED&C Excision
Inoperative tumors	Radiation therapy
Recurrent tumors	
Face	Mohs micrographic surgery
Trunk and extremities	Surgical excision
Pigmented	
Same treatment options as mentioned above for noduloulcerative lesions	
Superficial (Trunk)	
Primary	ED&C Cryotherapy (45-second freeze)
Recurrent	Surgical excision ED&C Mohs micrographic surgery

ED&C, electrodesiccation and curettage.

Electrodesiccation and Curettage

This modality is well suited to the treatment of superficial and nodular BCC. It is not appropriate and should not be used in the treatment of morpheaform BCC because of the indistinct margins. The tumor tissue is softer and more friable than the surrounding tissue. Initially, the bulk of the tumor is removed with the curette. The stroma and the surrounding dermis are then electrodesiccated. This cycle is repeated a maximum of two more times. After the procedure, the wound oozes serum before complete healing, which may take anywhere from 2 to 6 weeks.

TABLE 6 CRYOSURGERY

Advantages	Disadvantages
Quick procedure	Hypopigmentation
Lesser need for anesthesia	Prolonged healing period
Easy to use	High recurrence rate
Spares the patient a surgical procedure	Painful
	No tissue for margin control

Electrodesiccation and curettage is most suitable for small nodular and superficial cancers, and is not suitable for tumors that have extended beyond the dermis (Table 7). This form of therapy is not advocated for facial lesions, especially for tumors located in the facial creases such as the nasolabial fold and the preauricular skin. These biologic planes provide easy access for deep tumor invasion. The resultant cosmetic result with this modality is a circumscribed white patch that may be unacceptable to the younger population.

Radiation Therapy

Radiation therapy is best suited for elderly patients who are not suitable candidates for minor surgical procedures (Table 8). It is the procedure of choice in areas where preservation of normal surrounding tissue is of concern (e.g., around lips and eyes). Recurrence rates vary based on the size of the tumor being treated. BCCs located on the face that are less than 10 mm in diameter have an approximate 5% recurrence rate after 5-year follow-up, whereas tumors greater than 10 mm in diameter have a 5-year recurrence rate of 9.5%. This modality uses superficial x-rays administered in multiple divided doses over several weeks. This requires multiple outpatient visits, which may be difficult for some patients. In general, a total of 10 treatments is needed; this greatly reduces scarring, which was a common sequela of single-dose treatment. However, permanent epidermal atrophy, chronic radiation dermatitis, and the potential for delayed radiation-induced skin cancers preclude its use in the younger age group. Radiation therapy is contraindicated in the treatment of morpheaform BCC or recurrent BCC tumors, regardless of pathologic subtype.

Surgical Excision

Excision of the tumor produces a very elegant and unnoticeable scar and enables the pathologist to confirm the absence of tumor at the margins of the specimen (Table 9). An excisional margin of 3 to 4 mm of normal skin has been advocated to achieve the best cure rate while still allowing for a good cosmetic outcome.

Mohs Micrographic Surgery

Mohs surgery involves the removal of tumor by scalpel in sequential horizontal layers. Each tissue sample is frozen, stained, and microscopically examined. This

TABLE 7 ELECTRODESICCATION AND CURETTAGE

Advantages	Disadvantages
High cure rate	Scarring
Easy to perform	Hypopigmentation
Quick procedure	Prolonged healing
	No margin control

TABLE 8 RADIATION THERAPY

Advantages	Disadvantages
Spares surgical risks	Multiple treatment sessions and prolonged healing time
Elderly patient	Scar, radiation dermatitis
Inoperable tumor	No margin control

technique is the treatment of choice for BCCs that are more likely to recur based on anatomic location. This is especially true for those tumors with poorly defined margins. Repair of defects after Mohs surgery can be either immediate or delayed, and may be accomplished by either linear closure, adjacent tissue transfer, skin grafting, or healing by secondary intention.

Alternative Treatments

There are many ongoing investigational protocols to assess the effectiveness of alternate treatment modalities for BCC. One such protocol involves the administration of systemic retinoids to patients with multiple skin cancers. The use of isotretinoin in dosages of 2 mg/kg per day or etretinate at 1 mg/kg per day has been advocated. Although these regimens are not very effective in causing regression of existing tumors, studies have confirmed a significant reduction in new tumor formation in these patients.

Intralesional therapy with interferon is another modality that is under investigation. Interferon-α and interferon-γ have been found to be effective when administered three times per week over a 3-week period. A sustained-release formulation of interferon-α2b was developed in 1990; however, its long-term efficacy remains questionable. Side effects of treatment include a flu-like illness, nausea, and a mild increase in hepatic enzymes.

Photodynamic Therapy

This treatment modality involves the selective uptake of a photosensitizing agent by tumor cells. This is followed by exposure of tumor to laser light at specific wavelengths to allow for its destruction. The photosensitizing material is administered via intravenous injection. Topical agents are under study, however, and, with refinement, appear to hold great promise.

TABLE 9 SURGICAL EXCISION

Advantages	Disadvantages
Best cosmetic outcome	Incomplete margin control
High cure rate	

Follow-Up and Prognosis

Self-examination and regular follow-up are crucial in patients with BCC because they have a much higher propensity toward development of new skin cancers. Studies have shown that most patients with one BCC go on to acquire a second skin cancer within 5 years. Therefore, it is prudent to follow these patients for any sign of recurrence at the site of previous treatment, in addition to periodic full-skin examination. Strict sun avoidance should be emphasized.

The prognosis for most of those with BCC is extremely good because these are slowly growing tumors with rare potential for metastasis. However, if left untreated, these tumors can cause major destruction and result in the loss of vital structures.

Suggested Readings

Davis MM, Hanke CW, Zollinger TW, et al. Skin cancer in patients with chronic radiation dermatitis. *J Am Acad Dermatol* 1989;20:608–616.

Diwan R, Skouge JW. Basal cell carcinoma. *Curr Probl Dermatol* 1990;2:67–91.

Gupta AK, Cardella CJ, Haberman L. Cutaneous malignant neoplasms in patients with renal transplants. *Arch Dermatol* 1986;122:1288–1293.

Jacobs GH, Rippey JJ, Altini M. Prediction of aggressive behavior in basal cell carcinoma. *Cancer* 1982;49:533–537.

Miller SJ. Biology of basal cell carcinoma. *J Am Acad Dermatol* 1991;24:1–13.

Pollack SV, Goslen JB, Sheretz EF, et al. The biology of basal cell carcinoma: a review. *J Am Acad Dermatol* 1982;7:569–577.

Robinson JK. Risk of developing another basal cell carcinoma: a 5-year prospective study. *Cancer* 1987;60:118–120.

Robinson JK. What are adequate treatment and follow-up care for nonmelanoma cutaneous cancer? *Arch Dermatol* 1987;123:331–333.

Roenigk RK, Ratz JL, Bailin PL, et al. Trends in the presentation and treatment of basal cell carcinomas. *Journal of Dermatololgic Surgery and Oncology* 1986;12:860–865.

Rowe DE, Carroll RJ, Day CL. Long term recurrence rates on previously untreated basal cell carcinoma: implications for patient follow-up. *Journal of Dermatologic Surgery and Oncology* 1989;15:315–328.

Safai B, Good RA. Basal cell carcinoma with metastasis: review of the literature. *Arch Pathol Lab Med* 1977;101:327–331.

Schreiber MM, Moon TE, Fox SH, et al. The risk of developing nonmelanoma skin cancers. *J Am Acad Dermatol* 1990;23:1114–1118.

Sloane JP. The value of typing basal cell carcinomas in predicting recurrence after surgical excision. *Br J Dermatol* 1977;96:127–132.

Spiller WF, Spiller RF. Treatment of basal cell epithelioma by curettage and electrodesiccation. *J Am Acad Dermatol* 1984;11:808–814.

Zaynoun S, Lina AA, Shaib J, et al. The relationship of sun exposure and solar elastosis to basal cell carcinoma. *J Am Acad Dermatol* 1985;12:522–525.

CHAPTER 4

Squamous Cell Carcinoma

Epidemiology

Cutaneous squamous cell carcinoma (SCC) is a malignant neoplasm of the keratinizing cells of the epidermis. It is the second most common malignancy of the skin (after basal cell carcinoma [BCC]), accounting for approximately 20% of all skin cancers. There is currently an epidemic of SCC, with more than an estimated 100,000 new cases diagnosed each year in the United States alone. This accounts for approximately 2500 deaths annually. It is likely that the modern lifestyle preference for a tanned appearance, along with the depletion of the ozone layer, account for this continuing increased incidence of skin cancer.

Cutaneous SCC occurs most commonly in the elderly white population, with most patients in their sixth to seventh decade of life. There is an approximate 2:1 ratio of men to women. In blacks, SCC is much more common than BCC. SCC grows more rapidly than BCC. It is also more likely to invade underlying structures and to metastasize to distant body parts. The metastatic rate for SCC arising on sun-damaged skin is approximately 2% to 6%. This figure rises to approximately 10% for SCC involving the lip and 30% for SCC arising in scars.

Risk Factors

Ultraviolet (UV) radiation is the major risk factor for the development of cutaneous SCC in the white population (Table 1). These people usually have a poor tanning ability, fair skin, blond or reddish hair, blue eyes, and a Celtic background. It has been shown that the incidence of SCC significantly increases with proximity to the equator, emphasizing the role of UV radiation in the induction of nonmelanoma skin cancers. The areas of the body with the highest predilection

TABLE 1 RISK FACTORS FOR DEVELOPMENT OF SQUAMOUS CELL CARCINOMA

Chronic sun exposure
Fair skin/light hair
Cigarette smoking
Artificial tanning salons
Presence of actinic kertosis
Photochemotherapy (psoralens plus ultraviolet A)
Ionizing radiation
Chemical exposure (tar, arsenic)
Thermal burns/scars
Chronic inflammatory conditions
Immunosuppression
Human papillomavirus infection

for SCC—the scalp, face, and back of the hands—also correlate with areas of maximal UV exposure. Severe, blistering sunburns during childhood have also been shown to be an important etiologic factor. Artificial tanning booths are another important association.

Actinic keratoses are premalignant skin lesions that occur on sun-exposed areas such as the face, lower lip, and dorsum of hands, indicating extensive sun damage (Figs. 1–11). The risk of transformation to SCC is very low, probably less than 1% of cases. A lifetime risk of 12% for development of SCC in the presence of numerous actinic keratoses has also been reported.

Long-term use of photochemotherapy in the treatment of psoriasis by ingestion of psoralen, a photosensitizer, followed by exposure to UVA (psoralen plus UVA [PUVA]) is now a well-established predisposing factor to the development of SCC. In some studies, as much as a 30-fold increase in the incidence of SCC has been noted.

Early in the century, ionizing radiation was extensively used to treat skin cancer as well as a variety of benign skin conditions such as eczema and tinea. However, the association of this treatment modality with the development of cutaneous carcinoma was noted early. Total cumulative dose of ionizing radiation

(Text continues on page 79)

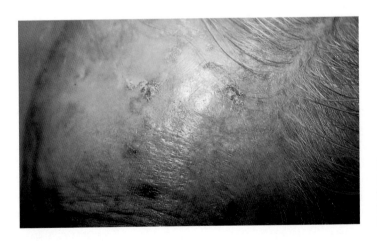

Figure 1

Multiple actinic keratoses on the frontal scalp with the characteristic rough, scaly, indurated appearance.

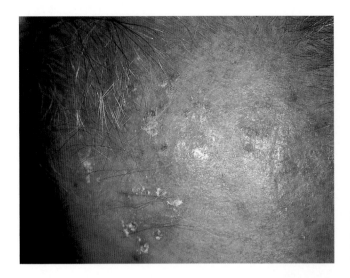

Figure 2

A close-up view of actinic keratoses scattered amid sun-damaged skin on the frontal scalp.

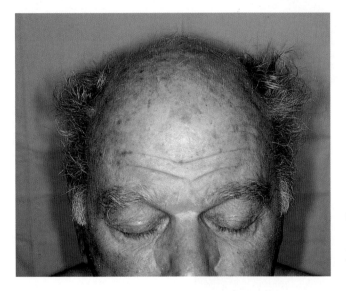

Figure 3

Multiple actinic keratoses. The face, scalp, lower lips, and dorsum of the hands are common sites of involvement.

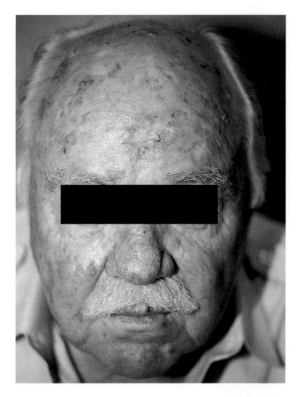

Figure 4

Multiple actinic keratoses. Chronic sun exposure is the major risk factor for development of these lesions.

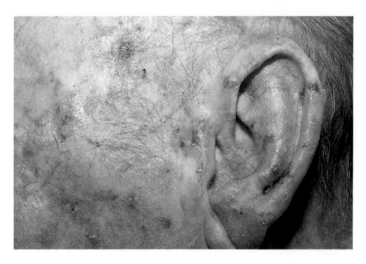

Figure 5

Multiple actinic keratoses. If left untreated, these tumors may progress to squamous cell carcinoma in 1% to 5% of cases.

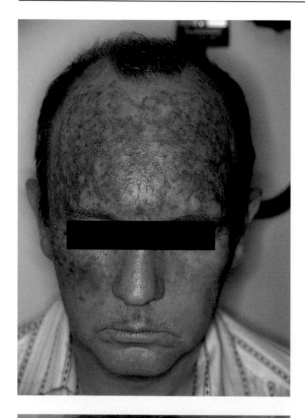

Figure 6

Patient with a preponderance of actinic keratoses after treatment with 5-fluorouracil cream. Note the inflammatory response of the skin.

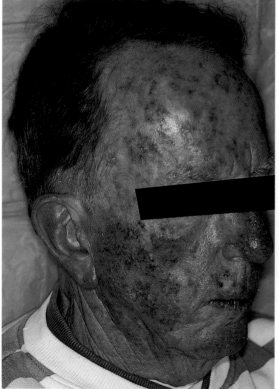

Figure 7

Patient with extensive sun damage and multiple actinic keratoses after treatment with 5-fluorouracil cream.

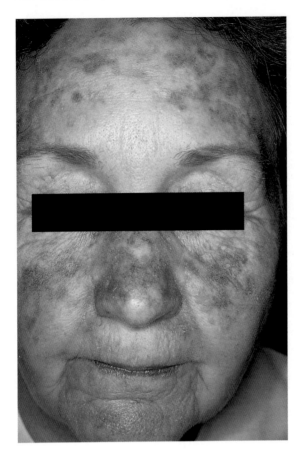

Figure 8

The inflammatory response gradually subsides after completion of treatment with 5-fluorouracil cream. This woman is 1 week post-treatment.

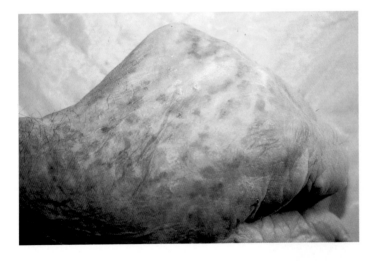

Figure 9

Multiple actinic keratoses, dorsum of left hand. The hypopigmented areas are the result of treatment with liquid nitrogen.

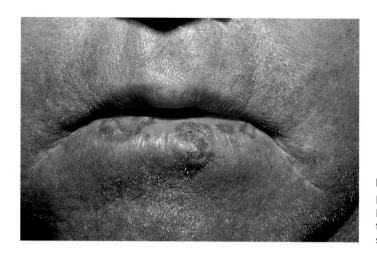

Figure 10

Hypertrophic actinic keratosis, lower lip. Biopsy showed that the tumor had not yet progressed to squamous cell carcinoma.

seems to be the predominant factor in the development of SCC. Chemical exposure to combusted tar, petroleum, and arsenic may also give rise to SCC. Smoking or chewing tobacco tobacco have both been linked to the development of SCC.

Inflammatory skin diseases may also develop into SCC. SCCs may arise in scars from thermal burns and leg ulcers, as well as in lesions of lichen planus, discoid lupus erythematosus, lichen sclerosus atrophicus, chronic osteomyelitis, and draining sinuses such as pilonidal sinus. In fact, scarring processes such as burns and leg ulcers are the most common predisposing conditions in the development of SCC in blacks. This is in contrast to whites, in whom UV light plays the major role.

It has been noted that immunosuppressed people have a higher rate of occurrence of SCC and a more aggressive disease progression. These include transplant recipients on immunosuppressive therapy as well as patients with lymphoma, leukemia, or human immunodeficiency virus infection. One study found a greater than 250-fold increase in the risk of SCC in renal transplant patients on immunosuppressive medication. In patients receiving immunosuppressive medication after renal transplantation, SCCs most commonly occur on the sun-exposed areas of the body. There is a delay between the initiation of immunosuppressive

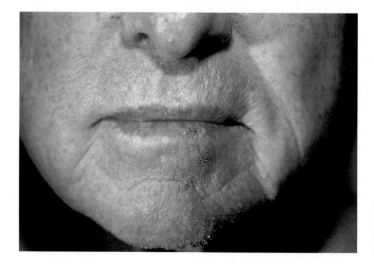

Figure 11

Actinic keratosis, lower lip. It is an indication of extensive sun damage.

medication and the onset of skin cancer of approximately 5 years. SCCs occur with a greater frequency than BCCs in immunosuppressed people. This is interesting, because there is a 4:1 ratio of BCC to SCC in the normal population.

Viral infection is another predisposing factor in the development of SCC. Certain strains of human papillomavirus (HPV), specifically types 16, 18, 31, and 33, are known causes of genital SCC. Fragments of HPV have been detected in SCCs of the vagina, anus, penis, vulva, and the digit. In contrast, SCCs arising on sun-exposed skin do not show evidence of infection with HPV.

As with BCC, genetic diseases such as xeroderma pigmentosum and oculocutaneous albinism render a person susceptible to development of SCCs in sun-exposed areas.

Pathogenesis

The precise mechanism of evolution of SCC is unknown. UV light, as already mentioned, is a major factor in its development. UVB has long been considered crucial in the induction of skin cancer. However, the hazardous effects of UVA are just being realized. UVB predisposes to SCC formation through two major mechanisms. First, UVB has been shown to have damaging effects on DNA. It induces the formation of DNA pyrimidine dimers in the keratinocytes, which result in specific DNA mutations in the cell. These characteristic mutations have been found in tumor cells of SCC. UV-induced DNA mutations are also found in tumor suppressor genes. The products of these genes are responsible for the regulation of the cell cycle. With any cellular damage, these genes become overexpressed and act to repair any mutation. The *p53* gene is an example of a tumor suppressor gene in which the characteristic UV-induced pyrimidine dimers are found. This mutated gene results in a nonfunctional protein that is unable to repair a mutated keratinocyte. This leads to uncontrolled regulation of the keratinocyte cell cycle with unlimited proliferation of the abnormal keratinocytes.

Ultraviolet B has also been proposed to induce skin cancer through interference with cellular immune mechanisms. UVB causes injury to the epidermal Langerhans cells, the key regulators of immunity in the skin. The Langerhans cells are then unable to process antigen and initiate a cascade of immune and inflammatory mediators. By interfering with the skin's immune function, UVB leads to a state of local immune tolerance and results in the skin's inability to limit tumor growth. This state of local immunosuppression is also highlighted by an increase in local T-suppressor cells with UV exposure.

Ultraviolet A is also crucial in the development of SCC. PUVA, a regimen mainly used in the treatment of psoriasis, is associated with the development of SCC. Psoriatic patients who are exposed to long-term PUVA are at a much higher risk for development of SCC.

Chemical carcinogenesis is another pathogenic mechanism in the formation of SCC. HPV is known to be associated with cervical cancer and has been found in certain cutaneous SCCs, mainly those of the genitalia and digits. It has been shown that certain characteristic fragments of this virus bind to the keratinocyte *p53* gene and interfere with its tumor suppressor function, which results in uncontrolled keratinocyte proliferation.

Clinical Features

Like BCC, SCC is most commonly found in sun-exposed areas. However, its pattern of distribution differs significantly from that of BCC. It most commonly occurs on the scalp and dorsum of the hands. BCC, in contrast, is rarely found in these locations. SCC begins as a small, erythematous, scaly, crusted patch. At this stage, there is atypia of the keratinocytes confined to the full thickness of the epidermis. This is known as SCC-*in-situ* or Bowen disease (Fig. 12). With time, the lesion may enlarge, with invasion of the atypical cells beyond the basement membrane into the dermis. This is termed *invasive SCC.* In some instances, this tumor is indistinguishable from an entity termed *keratoacanthoma.* Keratoacanthoma is clinically characterized as a suddenly appearing and rapidly growing, skin-colored to red nodule on sun-exposed skin with a central crater filled with a keratin plug (Figs. 13–23). Keratoacanthoma grows rapidly until it reaches a certain size, at which time it stops growing; it then begins slowly to resolve over the next few weeks to months, leaving behind a scar. An early SCC may also be confused with a hypertrophic actinic keratosis. Because these two entities are clinically indistinguishable, a shave biopsy must include the base of the specimen to make an accurate diagnosis.

A hypertrophic actinic keratosis is characterized by partial-thickness atypia of the epidermis with a thickened stratum corneum; SCC, however, is distinguished by epidermal atypia invading into the dermis (Figs. 24–49).

Some inflammatory and infectious disorders may be clinically mistaken for SCC. These include psoriasis, halogenoderma, and deep fungal infections such as

(Text continues on page 96)

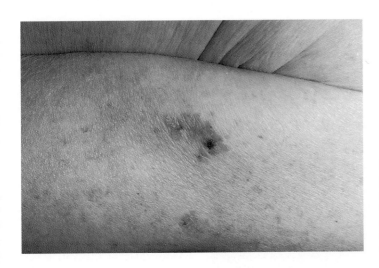

Figure 12

Bowen disease. This is squamous cell carcinoma confined to the epidermis. Appearing as an erythematous plaque, it may be mistaken for psoriasis or eczema.

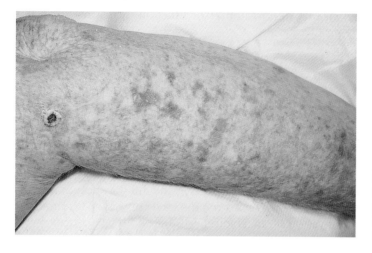

Figure 13
Multiple acinic keratoses on the arm. A hypertrophic actinic keratosis is present on the lateral aspect of the antecubital fossa.

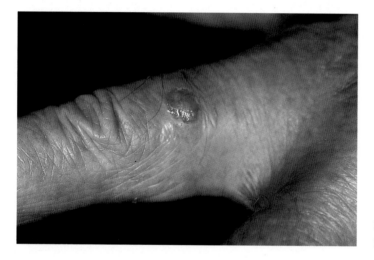

Figure 14
Bowen disease, right ring finger.

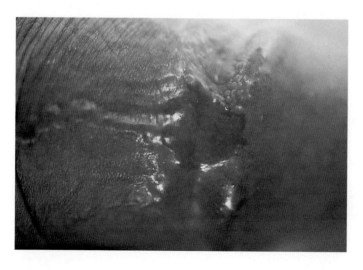

Figure 15
Erythroplasia of Queyrat, a synonym for Bowen disease occurring on the penis.

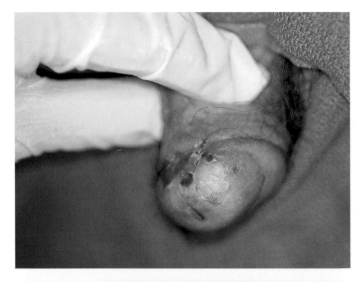

Figure 16
Erythroplasia of Queyrat. This tumor may respond to treatment with 5-fluorouracil cream.

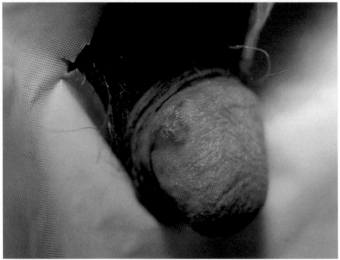

Figure 17
Erythroplasia of Queyrat.

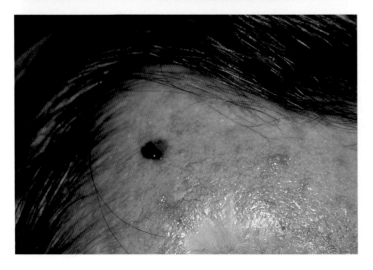

Figure 18
Keratoacanthoma. This lesion appeared suddenly, developing within weeks to months.

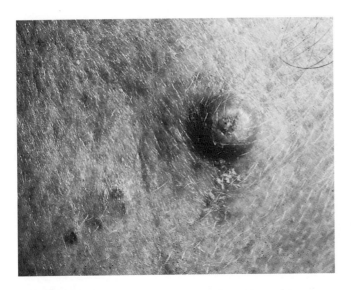

Figure 19

Keratoacanthoma. This lesion could easily be mistaken for squamous cell carcinoma.

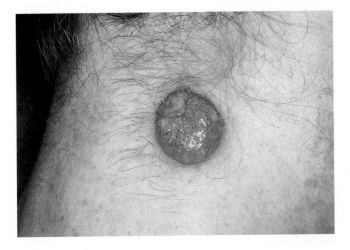

Figure 20

Keratoacanthoma. This is a benign epithelial neoplasm, but its fast growth rate could be rather alarming to the patient.

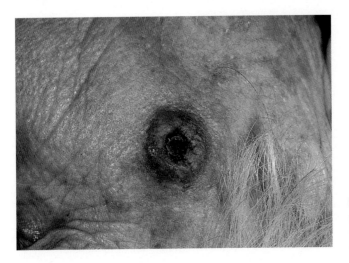

Figure 21

Keratoacanthoma. Note classic appearance as a firm, pink nodule with a keratotic center.

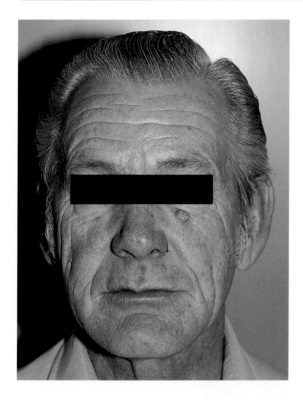

Figure 22

Keratoacanthoma, right cheek. Spontaneous regression is the rule with this tumor.

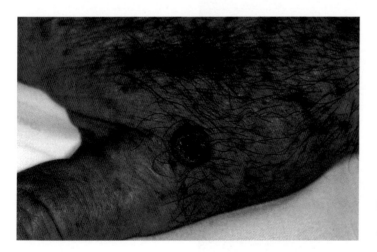

Figure 23

Keratoacanthoma, dorsum of the hand.

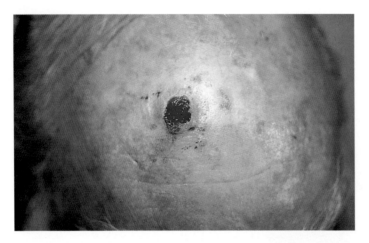

Figure 24
Squamous cell carcinoma, upper forehead. This nodule eventually ulcerated to its present form.

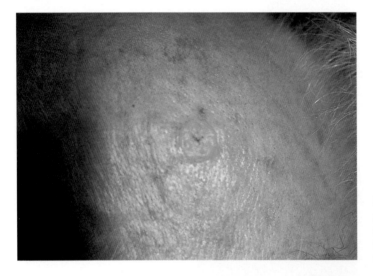

Figure 25
Squamous cell carcinoma, forehead. A shave biopsy confirmed the diagnosis in this well-circumscribed pink nodule.

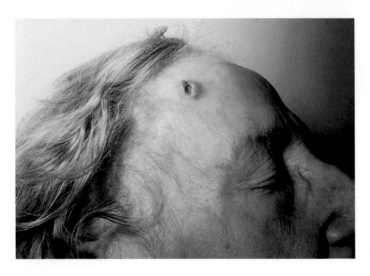

Figure 26
Squamous cell carcinoma. Superficial crusting is characteristic.

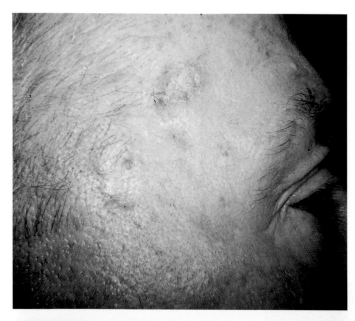

Figure 27

Squamous cell carcinoma, right temple.

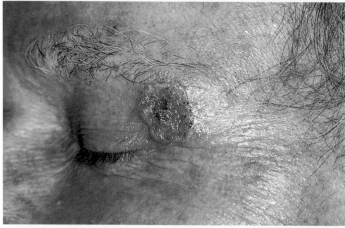

Figure 28

Squamous cell carcinoma, left lateral eye. Mohs surgery with extensive reconstruction of the defect was required.

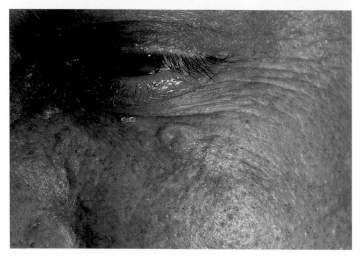

Figure 29

Squamous cell carcinoma, left lower eyelid skin.

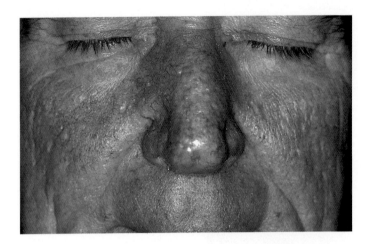

Figure 30
Squamous cell carcinoma of the nose.

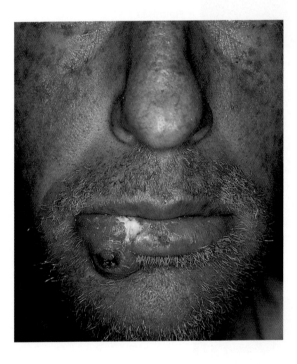

Figure 31
Squamous cell carcinoma, lower lip. Tumors on the lip have a much higher rate of metastasis, and aggressive intervention is a must.

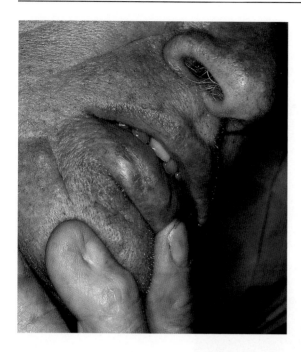

Figure 32

Squamous cell carcinoma, lower lip.

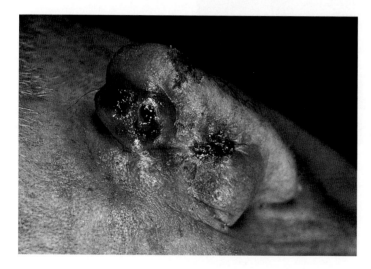

Figure 33

Squamous cell carcinoma. Tumors on the ear also have a higher risk of spread. Examination of lymph nodes with follow-up imaging studies indicated metastasis of the tumor in this patient.

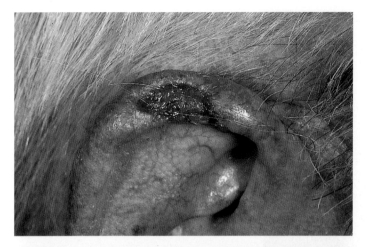

Figure 34

Squamous cell carcinoma. Patient presented to the clinic with the complaint of persistent ulceration on the ear.

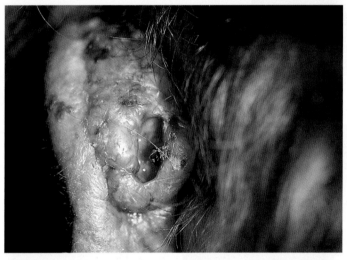

Figure 35

Advanced squamous cell carcinoma. Note the exudative crusted appearance.

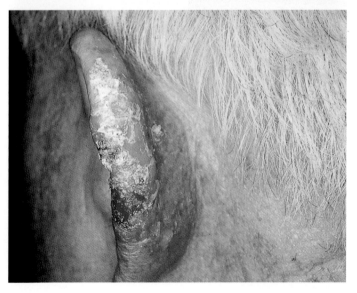

Figure 36

Squamous cell carcinoma, left helical rim. The ear is a common location for this tumor.

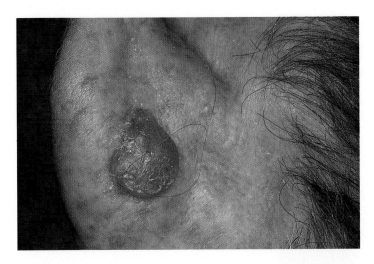

Figure 37

Squamous cell carcinoma, posterior ear.

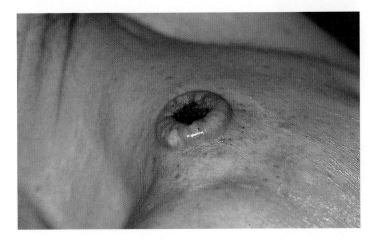

Figure 38

Squamous cell carcinoma arising in a persistent lesion of discoid lupus erythematosus. This tumor has a predilection for scars.

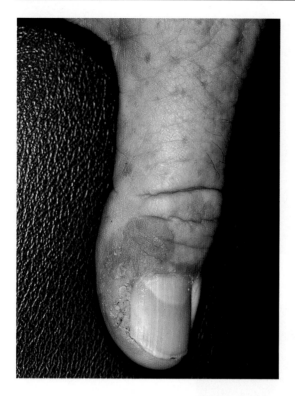

Figure 39
Squamous cell carcinoma, periungual region. This tumor was presumed to be a wart and treated with liquid nitrogen on multiple occasions. Eventual biopsy led to the correct diagnosis.

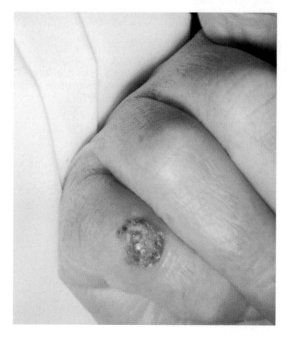

Figure 40
Squamous cell carcinoma, dorsum of the finger.

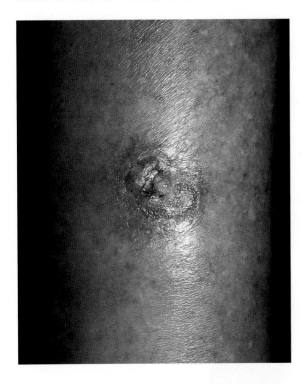

Figure 41
Squamous cell carcinoma on the leg. All cutaneous sites are susceptible.

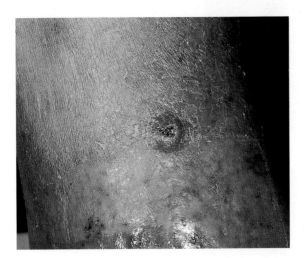

Figure 42
Squamous cell carcinoma. This is an early tumor in a patient with stasis dermatitis.

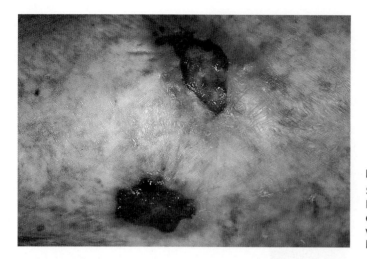

Figure 43

Squamous cell carcinoma, lower leg. This tumor should be considered for any nonhealing, persistent venous stasis ulceration on the lower legs.

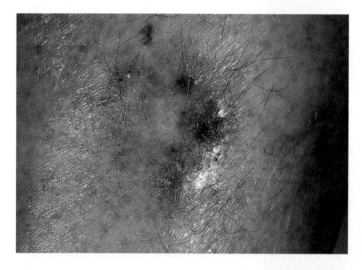

Figure 44

Squamous cell carcinoma. This tumor has a tendency toward crusting.

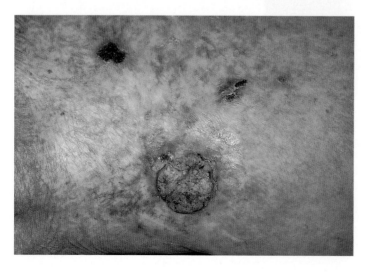

Figure 45

Squamous cell carcinoma. This is a vegetative nodule on the leg.

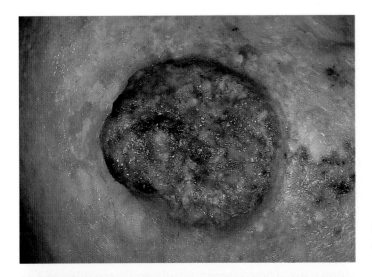

Figure 46

Squamous cell carcinoma. This large nodule has been ignored.

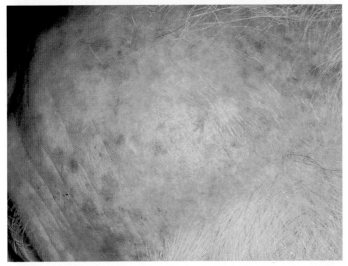

Figure 47

Multiple actinic keratoses on the forehead and scalp.

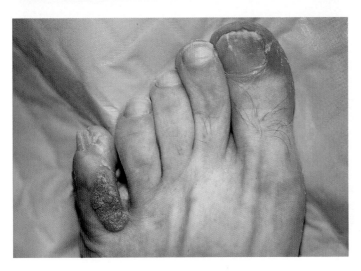

Figure 48

Squamous cell carcinoma in the periungual area.

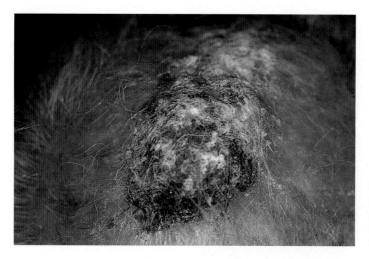

Figure 49

Large crusted nodule on the scalp. This clinical presentation is almost pathognomonic for squamous cell carcinoma.

sporotrichosis and blastomycosis. These diseases histologically resemble SCC as well. The architectural pattern of these conditions shows epithelial hyperplasia similar to that seen in SCC. However, there is an absence of both keratinocyte atypia and atypical mitotic figures, which are commonly seen in SCC.

Histopathology

Squamous cell carcinoma is histologically characterized by a downgrowth of atypical keratinocytes into the dermis (Figs. 50–59). Atypia involving only the full thickness of the epidermis is known as SCC-*in-situ* or Bowen disease. The degree of differentiation of the keratinocytes has been used to grade SCC. This is known as the Broder's classification, and involves four grades of cell differentiation. Grade

(Text continues on page 100)

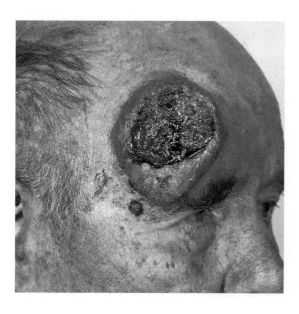

Figure 50

Advanced squamous cell carcinoma. On surgical excision of the tumor, perineural as well as bone involvement was noted.

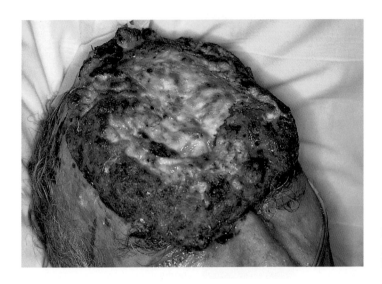

Figure 51

Extensive squamous cell carcinoma in a bedridden patient.

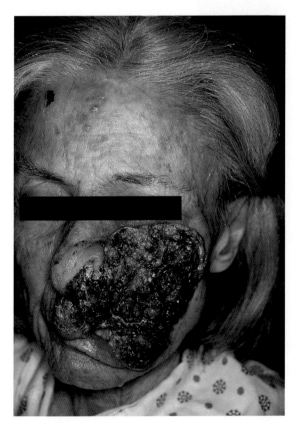

Figure 52

Extensive squamous cell carcinoma. This patient later died of tumor metastasis.

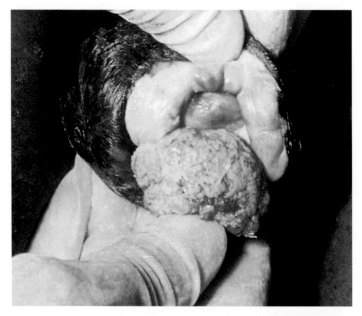

Figure 53

Squamous cell carcinoma of the penis.

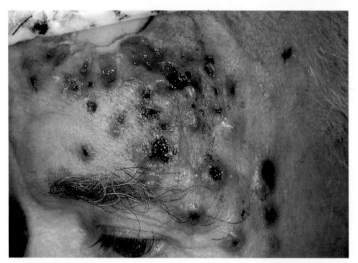

Figure 54

Metastatic cutaneous squamous cell carcinoma. At this stage, prognosis is extremely poor.

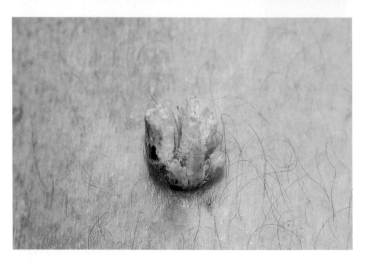

Figure 55

Cutaneous horn. A deep shave biopsy showed squamous cell carcinoma at the base of the tumor.

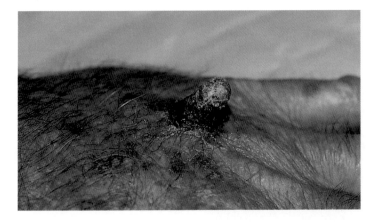

Figure 56

A hypertrophic actinic keratosis that was left untreated. A shave biopsy on presentation showed squamous cell carcinoma at the base of the tumor.

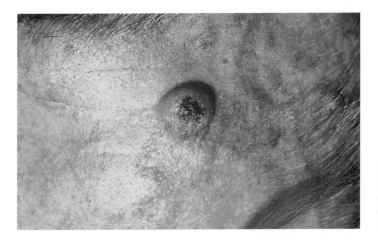

Figure 57

Keratoacanthoma. It is important to be able to differentiate this tumor from squamous cell carcinoma.

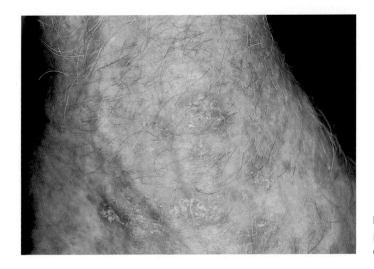

Figure 58

Multiple actinic keratoses on the dorsum of the hand.

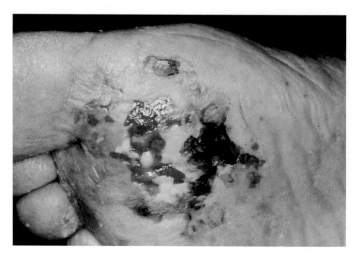

Figure 59
Squamous cell carcinoma on plantar aspect of the feet.

1 is considered well-differentiated carcinoma, whereas grade 4 is poorly differentiated SCC. It is known that well-differentiated SCC has a much lower incidence of deep invasion and therefore is associated with a better prognosis. The poorly differentiated pattern is associated with an increased rate of invasion and metastasis, and may histologically mimic other entities such as malignant melanoma, dermatofibrosarcoma protuberans, and atypical fibroxanthoma.

Serial immunohistochemical stains may be needed to differentiate these different types of tumors. Poorly differentiated SCC stains positively with monoclonal antibodies directed against cytokeratin. Electron microscopy can also aid in making an accurate diagnosis of poorly differentiated SCC by positive identification of desmosomes (cell bridges) and intracellular keratin filaments.

Treatment

Many different treatment modalities may be used to treat SCC (Table 2). These include electrodesiccation and curettage (ED&C), cryotherapy, radiation therapy, surgical excision, Mohs micrographic surgery, and carbon dioxide laser destruction. Treatment decisions should be based on clinical and histologic parameters, including the size and location of the lesion, its degree of cellular differentiation, its depth of invasion, and the presence of perineural invasion (Table 3).

**TABLE 2 TREATMENT MODALITIES
FOR SQUAMOUS CELL CARCINOMA**

Electrodesiccation and curettage
Cryotherapy
Radiation therapy
Surgical excision
Mohs micrographic surgery
Photodynamic therapy

TABLE 3 FACTORS INVOLVED IN CHOOSING THE APPROPRIATE TREATMENT MODALITY FOR SQUAMOUS CELL CARCINOMA

Clinical Parameters
    Patient's age
    Health status
    Anatomic location
    Primary versus recurrent tumor
    Size of tumor

Histologic Parameters
    Degree of differentiation of tumor cells
    Degree of invasion
    Presence of perineural spread or lymphatic invasion

Another important clinical parameter to consider is the location of the tumor. Sun-induced SCC has a lower rate of metastasis than SCC that develops in a setting of chronic inflammation, scarring, or radiation dermatitis. It has been shown that tumors on the lips, ears, and nose are at a much higher risk for spread. These tumors should ideally be treated with a modality that offers evidence for tumor-free margins. Recurrent SCC (tumor that recurs after original treatment) is much more aggressive, and therefore has a higher metastatic rate (Table 4).

The size of tumor is another important factor to be considered. It has been shown that tumors that exceed 2 cm in diameter are more likely to recur and metastasize, and thus should be treated more aggressively.

The increased incidence and aggressiveness of SCC in immunocompromised patients is well known. Studies have shown that transplant recipients on immunosuppressive medication as well as those with acquired immunodeficiency syndrome and lymphoma are at a higher risk for metastasis and death (Table 5).

Histologic parameters that determine therapy include the degree of differentiation, depth of invasion, and the presence of perineural involvement (Table 6). Well-differentiated SCC has a better prognosis than poorly differentiated tumors. Poorly differentiated SCC behaves aggressively and has a higher rate of recurrence and metastasis. Although it is less likely to spread, the capability of well-differentiated SCC to metastasize has been well documented. With regard to the depth of invasion, those tumors that penetrate into the papillary dermis have a much lower rate of recurrence and metastasis than tumors that invade into the deep dermis and subcutaneous fat. Patients with perineural involvement are at higher risk for local recurrence as well as spread of the tumor. These patients should be treated aggressively.

If a diagnosis of SCC is suspected, the status of local lymph nodes draining the tumor should be evaluated. The presence of any clinically palpable nodes may

TABLE 4 RISK FACTORS FOR INCREASED AGGRESSIVENESS OF SQUAMOUS CELL CARCINOMA

Tumor >2 cm
Tumor in scar
Immunosuppressed patient
Histologic study shows poorly differentiated tumor or evidence of perineural invasion

TABLE 5 SQUAMOUS CELL CARCINOMA IN TRANSPLANT PATIENTS

Metastasis	6.6%
Mortality	5.4%

be a sign of metastasis, and requires a careful work-up through a multidisciplinary approach.

Electrodesiccation and Curettage

This treatment modality is reserved for destruction of SCC-*in-situ* (Bowen disease) or small, recurrent, superficially invasive SCC of the trunk. This technique is fast and easy to perform, but in addition to its unsightly cosmetic outcome, no histologic margins are available to ensure tumor-free resection. This makes the close clinical follow-up of patients with SCC even more significant in patients treated with this technique. ED&C should not be used for tumors on the face because there may be extension of tumor cells deep along the hair follicles, beyond the reach of the curette. This technique is also unacceptable for "high-risk'" SCCs because of the greater possibility of recurrence and metastasis.

Cryosurgery

Cryosurgery is routinely used in the treatment of actinic keratosis. This technique, however, should not be used to treat SCC unless the operator is properly skilled in the use of thermocouples and cryoprobes with the liquid nitrogen spray unit. (Thermocouples and cryoprobes are instruments that are inserted into the base of the tumor to measure accurately the desired tumoricidal temperature.) Cotton-tipped applicators dipped in liquid nitrogen are absolutely ineffective in treating SCC. Because this technique offers no histologic margin control, pretreatment biopsies are a must to ensure that the tumor is superficial and well differentiated. In addition, cryotherapy should be used only in small tumors that are well demarcated and located on the trunk. If the lesions are selected appropriately, treatment of SCC with cryotherapy can be highly successful. Many studies have reported cure rates of greater than 95% using this modality. During treatment, it is important to include a rim of normal tissue beyond the clinically visible margins

TABLE 6 LIKELIHOOD OF METASTASIS OF SQUAMOUS CELL CARCINOMA BASED ON LOCATION

Location	Likelihood (%)
Lip	10
Temple	36
Ear	10
Hand	18
Nose	8–27
Leg	13

of the tumor. The patient should be advised that after treatment, a painful, blood-tinged, oozing blister may form. There is an approximate 2- to 4-week healing period depending on the duration and depth of the freeze. This eventuates in an atrophic, hypopigmented scar.

Carbon Dioxide Laser

The carbon dioxide laser may be used in its focused mode to excise SCC. Use of the laser allows for an accurate and cosmetic destruction of the tissue in a bloodless fashion because the laser seals small blood vessels during treatment. It not only provides a better cosmetic outcome than ED&C or cryotherapy, but it allows for margin control by histopathologic evaluation. The major disadvantage of this technique is the increased cost. Mainstream use of this modality is unlikely because it does not offer significant advantages over standard excision. Tumors involving the nail bed or the penis have responded well to carbon dioxide laser therapy.

Radiation Therapy

Although seldom used in the treatment of primary SCC, radiation therapy is an alternative that offers a greater than 90% cure rate when used in the treatment of appropriately selected patients. It is mainly used in elderly patients with multiple medical problems in whom surgery is a relative contraindication. It may also be used as palliative therapy in patients with inoperable tumors. Because radiation does not destroy normal tissue when administered appropriately, it is especially useful in the treatment of tumors in anatomically sensitive locations such as the periocular area. Radiation treatment is usually contraindicated in patients younger than 55 years of age because there is a slightly increased risk of induction of a second skin cancer. The treatment is divided into 10 to 15 doses, which requires multiple office visits. The particular features of the tumor are taken into consideration when deciding on the appropriate treatment regimen; for example, well-differentiated SCC requires a larger dose of radiation than poorly differentiated tumors. Although the immediate cosmetic result after treatment may be good, it worsens over time, with development of chronic radiation dermatitis. The treated site becomes atrophic and hypopigmented with telangiectatic vessels coursing through it.

5-Fluorouracil

Topical 5-fluorouracil has been successfully used in treating patients with extensive actinic keratoses (see Figs. 7 and 8). The 5% ointment has been found to be most appropriate in treating superficial lesions of Bowen disease. It offers the advantage of a noninvasive treatment option in a patient who is not a surgical candidate and who is unwilling to undergo other destructive modalities. Prolonged treatment for up to 16 weeks is necessary to achieve resolution of tumor. Close clinical follow-up to assess for recurrence of the tumor is a necessity. Because of its variable level of penetration, 5-fluorouracil should not be used in treating SCC.

It offers no histologic margins, and the deep component of the tumor may be left behind, resulting in the subclinical spread of the tumor. This modality is not indicated in the treatment of invasive SCC.

Surgical Excision

Surgical excision is the standard modality used in the treatment of SCC. It allows for histologic control of margins, rapid healing, and an excellent cosmetic result if performed appropriately. When considering excisional margins, the specific features of the tumor should be taken into account. For well-differentiated tumors that are less than 2 cm in size, studies have shown that 4-mm margins of normal tissue around the visible borders of the tumor allow for the lowest recurrence rates while still resulting in a good cosmetic outcome.

For larger or more aggressive tumors, the clinical margin should be increased accordingly. When surgery is performed appropriately, impressive 5-year cure rates of 98% have been reported. This is a time-consuming technique that requires some expertise to achieve optimal results. It also spares normal tissue and may not be appropriate in treating patients with heavily sun-damaged skin and multiple skin cancers.

Mohs Micrographic Surgery

Microscopically controlled excision with the aid of Mohs micrographic surgery is considered the gold standard in treating "high-risk'" SCC. This modality offers a cure rate in the order of 99% for primary cutaneous SCC and 95% for recurrent tumors. It permits the complete removal of the tumor during surgery while allowing for maximal preservation of normal tissue. Although time consuming and tedious, when available, no other treatment modality should be considered for high-risk tumors. These include ill-defined, large, poorly differentiated, deeply invasive, or recurrent tumors. This technique is especially indicated for tumors located in anatomic areas at high risk for recurrence (i.e., ear, lip, nose, and periocular area). If deemed appropriate, postoperative radiation may be considered for those patients at high risk for metastasis.

Alternative Treatments

Photodynamic therapy, interferon, interleukin-2, chemotherapy, and retinoids are alternative modalities under exploration for the treatment of SCC.

TABLE 7 INDICATORS OF A POORER PROGNOSIS IN SQUAMOUS CELL CARCINOMA

Tumor >2 cm
Tumor arising in previously irradiated area
Tumor arising in a previous scar
Deep tumors
Perineural invasion
Immunosuppressed patient

TABLE 8 HISTOLOGIC INDICATORS OF POORER PROGNOSIS IN SQUAMOUS CELL CARCINOMA

Poorly differentiated
Deep invasion
Thick tumor
Perineural spread or lymphatic involvement

Follow-Up and Prognosis

It is imperative that patients with SCC have regular skin and lymph node examination to check for any evidence of local recurrence, lymph node metastasis, or new disease. There should also be a low threshold for biopsy of any suspect skin lesions (Table 7). Strict sun avoidance, along with the regular use of broad-spectrum sunscreens, is a must. The prognosis of sun-induced primary SCC is in general very good, with a low risk of metastasis if treated early. However, large, invasive tumors and those located in high-risk anatomic sites need to be treated aggressively because of their high metastatic rate. The factors associated with an increased tendency for SCC to metastasize include site, depth of invasion, histologic differentiation, rapidity of growth, anatomic site, presence of immunosuppression, evidence of neurotropism, and recurrence of the tumor after treatment (Table 8).

Suggested Readings

Brownstein MH, Rabinowitz AD. The precursors of cutaneous squamous cell carcinoma. *Int J Dermatol* 1979;18:1–16.

Cottel WI. Perineural invasion by squamous cell carcinoma. *Journal of Dermatologic and Surgical Oncology* 1982;8:589–600.

Dzubow LM, Rigel DS, Robins P. Risk factors for local recurrence of primary cutaneous squamous cell carcinomas: treatment by microscopically controlled excision. *Arch Dermatol* 1982;118:900–902.

Epstein E. Metastases of sun-induced squamous cell carcinoma. *Journal of Dermatologic and Surgical Oncology* 1984;10:418.

Glass AG, Hoover RN. The emerging epidemic of melanoma and squamous cell carcinoma. *JAMA* 1989;262:2097–2100.

Honeycutt WM, Jansen T. Treatment of squamous cell carcinoma of the skin. *Arch Dermatol* 1973;108:670–672.

Jones RR. Ozone depletion and cancer risk. *Lancet* 1987;2:443–446.

Koo KC, Carter RL O'Brien CJ, et al. Prognostic implications of perineural spread in squamous carcinomas of the head and neck. *Laryngoscope* 1986;96:1145–1148.

Marks R, Rennie G, Selwood T. The relationship of basal cell carcinomas and squamous cell carcinomas to solar keratoses. *Arch Dermatol* 1988;124:1039–1042.

Wilson SM, Phillips JM, Hawk JC. Metastases from squamous cell carcinoma of the skin. *J S C Med Assoc* 1990;86:311–314.

CHAPTER 5

MALIGNANT MELANOMA

Epidemiology

The incidence of cutaneous melanoma is growing at a rate faster than any other human malignancy. In the United States alone, there is a 7% yearly increase in the incidence of melanoma, and by the year 2000, it has been projected that this malignancy will have developed in 1 in every 75 to 90 Americans. In 1935, only 1 per 1500 people would acquire melanoma over his or her lifetime. The American Cancer Society has estimated that 32,000 new cases of melanoma were diagnosed in the United States in 1994, and 6000 people died of the disease. An estimated 38,000 cases of invasive melanoma and 30,000 to 50,000 new cases of melanoma-in-situ were diagnosed in the United States in 1996. This phenomenon is not restricted to the United States alone. The incidence of melanoma has doubled in Australia and Scandinavia since the late 1980s. In Australia, melanoma has certainly reached epidemic proportions, with 1 in every 17 women and 1 in every 14 men acquiring melanoma over his or her lifetime.

Melanoma is rare in childhood and adolescence. When it does occur in this age group, it mostly arises in giant congenital nevi (Figs. 1–12). Melanoma is seen more frequently in the third decade and becomes most preponderant in the fourth and fifth decades. The most common site of the tumor in women is the leg; the back is most commonly afflicted in men.

Risk Factors

A number of factors seem to be responsible for the increased incidence of melanoma. The greatest impact has come from lifestyle changes resulting in increased recreational exposure of whites to ultraviolet (UV) light (Table 1). There

(Text continues on page 112)

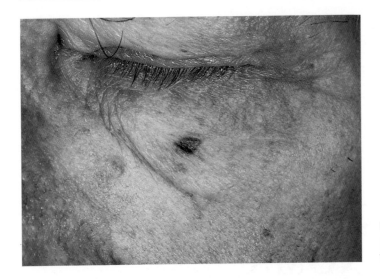

Figure 1
Melanocytic nevus, a benign entity.

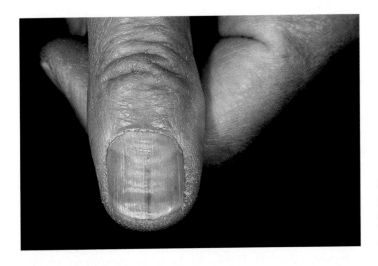

Figure 2
Melanonychia striata, an acquired pigmented band on the fingernail. Biopsy of the nail bed showed no sign of malignancy.

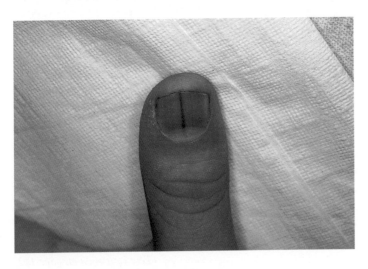

Figure 3
Junctional nevus of the nail bed.

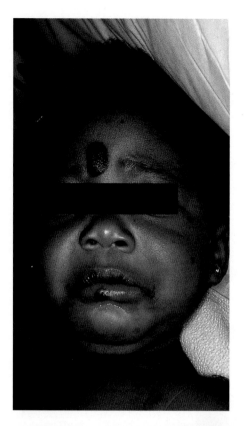

Figure 4
Multiple congenital nevi in an otherwise healthy child.

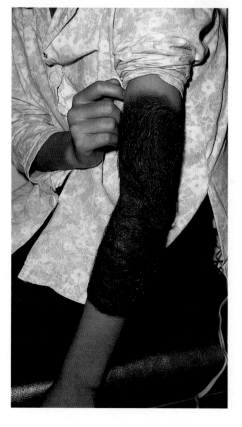

Figure 5
Congenital hairy nevus. This lesion is present at birth.

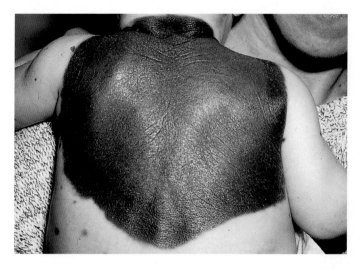

Figure 6
Congenital nevus, upper back.

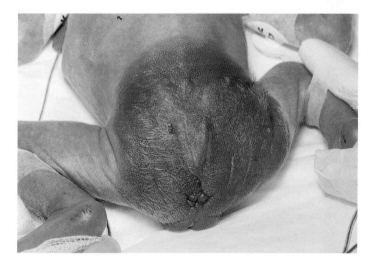

Figure 7
Congenital nevus. Special attention should be paid to any localized nodules or nonhealing erosions.

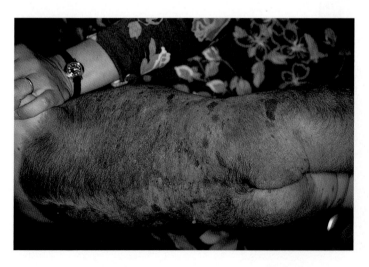

Figure 8
Extensive congenital nevus covering most of the body.

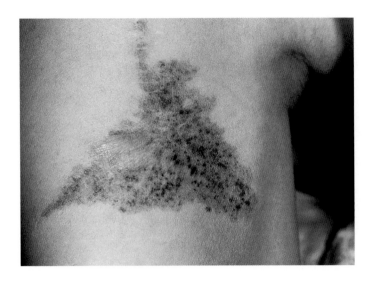

Figure 9

Nevus spilus. There is a patch with multiple, small, darker-pigmented macules within the lesion.

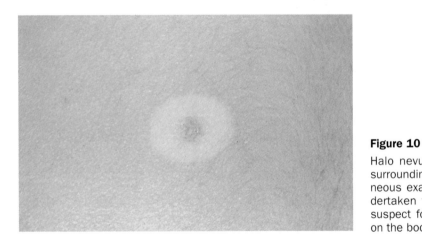

Figure 10

Halo nevus, a lightening of skin surrounding the nevus. A full cutaneous examination should be undertaken to rule out any lesions suspect for melanoma elsewhere on the body.

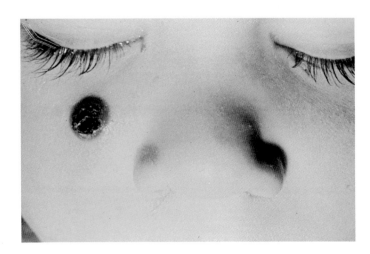

Figure 11

Spitz nevus, a benign lesion that occurs more commonly in children.

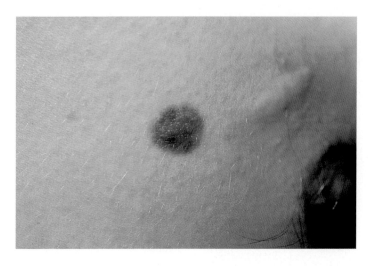

Figure 12
Atypical nevus. Note the atypical brownish pigmentation in the lesion.

TABLE 1 ROLE OF SUN EXPOSURE IN MELANOMA

Latitude-dependent increase in melanoma; increased numbers closer to equator
Intermittent intense sun exposure is correlated to the risk for development of melanoma
Increased risk with history of multiple sunburns
Increased risk of melanoma in those living in sunny climates at a young age
Increased risk of melanoma in those with fair skin
Increased risk of melanoma in whites
UV exposure and risk of melanoma not linearly correlated
Body regions with highest UV exposure not at highest risk for melanoma
Dark-skinned races more frequently have melanomas on palmar/plantar surfaces, subungual
    regions, and mucosa

UV, ultraviolet.

TABLE 2 SKIN PHOTOTYPES

I	Always burns, never tans
II	Easily burns, rarely tans
III	Sometimes burns, usually tans
IV	Rarely burns, always tans
V	Always tans; moderately pigmented (brown)
VI	Always tans; darkly pigmented (black)

TABLE 3 FAMILIAL DYSPLASTIC NEVUS SYNDROME

Also called the familial atypical mole–melanoma syndrome
Patients have large number of (>50) atypical-appearing nevi
This trait is inherited in an autosomal dominant fashion, although it is only variably expressed
Linked to chromosome 9p
One or more first-degree relatives have melanoma
Lifetime risk for development of melanoma approaches 100% in those affected
Melanoma develops at an average age of 33 years; average age for the general population is 54
   years

are a multitude of studies supporting this fact. Among whites, melanoma incidence and mortality inversely correlate with the distance from the equator. The
migration of light-skinned people to areas of intense sun exposure, for which they
are poorly adapted, has left their descendants at high risk for melanoma. An ideal
example is Queensland, Australia, which is mostly inhabited by people of Celtic
descent from Ireland and Scotland. The response pattern of the skin to UV radiation is thus an important determinant of risk. Although darker-skinned people do
acquire melanoma, whites are at a far greater risk (Table 2).

The age at which exposure to intense UV radiation takes place also seems to
be particularly significant. One study showed that intense sun exposure during the
teenage years conveyed the greatest risk. In another study, it was shown that people who migrated to sunny climates at a young age have a higher risk for development of melanoma than their older counterparts.

The risk for melanoma is also greater for areas of intense intermittent sun exposure. This would explain the much higher incidence of melanoma on the legs
of women and on the backs of men rather than on the continually exposed skin of
the head and neck. It would also explain the much higher incidence of melanoma
in white-collar workers of higher socioeconomic status. These people tend to va-
cation in a warm climate and have an intense periodic exposure to UV rays on an
intermittent basis.

There is strong evidence for a genetic predisposition toward development of
melanoma. In certain families, members are afflicted with large numbers of clinically atypical-appearing nevi (Tables 3 and 4). These nevi develop in the first or
second decade and are much larger than usual. This condition, termed "hereditary dysplastic nevus syndrome," places the members at a greatly increased risk for
melanoma. In fact, if a close relative has had melanoma, the person has a 50%
chance of acquiring melanoma over his or her lifetime. If two or more close relatives have had melanoma, the risk approaches 100%. Gene mapping studies have
mapped a "melanoma susceptibility gene" to the short arm of chromosome nine.

People with multiple atypical nevi have been categorized by some as having
"dysplastic nevus syndrome." This is a controversial topic, but it appears that these

TABLE 4 CLASSIFICATION OF BENIGN NEVI

Junctional nevi
Compound nevi
Intradermal nevi

TABLE 5 MELANOMA RISK

Risk Factor	Risk[a]
FAMM syndrome with previous melanoma	500
FAMM syndrome with atypical nevi but no previous melanoma	150
Atypical nevi	7–20
Numerous common nevi	5–65
Previous melanoma	9

[a] Times over the general population.

FAMM, familial atypical mole–melanoma.

people are at a higher risk for development of melanoma than the general population, although the risk is much lower than in those with the familial syndrome (Table 5).

In one well publicized study, attempts to isolate risk factors for melanoma through multivariate analysis identified six factors that were most likely to influence the emergence of melanoma. These risk factors included a history of 3 or more years in an outdoor summer job as a teenager, history of actinic keratoses, blond or red hair, a family history of melanoma, three or more blistering sunburns before the age of 20 years, and higher-than-average freckling on the upper back. If one or two risk factors were present, the probability for the development of melanoma was increased three- to fivefold over the general population. If three or more risk factors were present, the relative risk was increased by 20-fold.

A personal history of melanoma is another risk factor for the development of melanoma. In fact, these people have a ninefold increased risk for development of a second, independent lesion over the general population.

Immunosuppressed patients are another population requiring close monitoring. Although not as dramatic as the increase in incidence of squamous cell carcinoma, an increase in the incidence of melanoma in transplant recipients has been well documented. Patients carrying the human immunodeficiency virus are also at a higher risk, although this risk is not as pronounced (Table 6).

Finally, it is important to point out that melanoma affects both sexes equally. Hormonal factors do not appear to have any influence in the development of melanoma.

TABLE 6 FOLLOW-UP GUIDELINES FOR PATIENTS WITH MELANOMA

Ten-year disease-free interval does not constitute a cure. Patients must have annual follow-up examinations for life.

Patients with "thicker" melanomas should be examined at more frequent intervals during the first few years after diagnosis than patients with thinner melanomas.

All melanoma patients should be examined at least annually for life because of their greater likelihood for development of new primary melanomas or a recurrence of their original lesion.

Immunosuppressed patients, patients with atypical mole syndrome, and patients with xeroderma pigmentosum should be examined more frequently.

Pathogenesis

Intensive research has been aimed at delineating the reasons for the progression of benign nevus cells to the malignant form. Thus far, the following three mechanisms have been found to account for tumor progression: mutations of protooncogenes, mutations of tumor suppressor genes, and structural changes in the DNA.

Melanoma most commonly arises at the site of normal-appearing skin (70% of cases), and arises at the site of a previously existing nevus in the remaining 30% of cases. Superficial spreading melanoma, a subtype of melanoma that is most commonly seen in younger people, is most commonly seen in association with melanocytic nevi. Sunlight exposure at an early age induces the proliferation of nevus cells, which clinically manifest as a melanocytic nevi. This is considered the first stage in the development of melanoma. From there on, intermittent overexposure to the sun is believed to promote further progression toward cancer. This correlates with the high incidence of this form of melanoma in the younger population, with a diminishing incidence in older age groups. In contrast, lentigo maligna melanoma, another subtype of melanoma, continually increases in incidence with age. Cumulative sun exposure accounts for repeated damage to the DNA of the melanocytes, which eventuates in the formation of melanoma.

Genetic factors play a large part in the pathogenesis of melanoma. Hair and skin color, the host's response to UV radiation, and the ability to repair damage to DNA are all genetically determined. For example, patients with xeroderma pigmentosum have a hereditary defect in their ability to repair damages to DNA. These patients have a several thousandfold increase in the incidence of melanoma over the general population.

Future research may show that oncogenes and tumor suppressor genes play a prominent role in the pathogenesis of melanoma. Oncogenes are mutant forms of protooncogenes, portions of DNA concerned with normal cellular growth. A structural alteration of these genes through a mutation may lead to uncontrolled growth and differentiation. Tumor suppressor genes may also be altered such that on exposure to a carcinogen, there is a rapid and accelerated development of tumor.

Clinical Features

Because of its accessibility to visual examination, melanoma may be diagnosed and treated at an early stage. Regardless of subtype, all melanomas present as a changing pigmented lesion (Table 7). The mnemonic, ABCDE—referring to **A**symmetry, **B**order irregularity, **C**olor variegation, **D**iameter greater than 7 mm, and **El**evation above the skin surface—has been very successful in pubic education campaigns (Table 8).

Other clinical features should be taken into consideration when evaluating a pigmented lesion. Pruritus, tenderness, and oozing or bleeding may all be accompanying symptoms. Table 9 lists common distal sites of metastatic melanoma.

Most melanomas arise *de novo* in normal skin. Approximately 30% seem to arise in a preexisting nevus.

TABLE 7 PIGMENTED LESIONS SIMULATING MELANOMA

Recurrent nevus: When a melanocytic nevus has been removed incompletely by a shave biopsy. Recurs with irregular borders and irregular pigmentation.

Spitz nevus: Pink, occasionally brown-pigmented, raised lesion, usually on the face or leg; often arises in infancy or childhood.

Halo nevus: Melanocytic nevus surrounded by a symmetric zone of depigmentation. Commonly occurs in adolescents, especially on trunk. Usually more than one nevus is affected at one time.

Congenital nevus: Present at birth, grows proportionately with patient. Color ranges from tan to black. Melanoma may arise in these lesions, especially the larger ones.

Blue nevus: Seen frequently early in life; bluish, dome-shaped, and smooth-surfaced.

Pyogenic granuloma: Exbuerant, fleshy granulation tissue usually resulting from trauma. Usually red to brown in color, solitary. Bleeds easily. Usually seen in children and pregnant women.

Angiokeratoma: A red papule with a thick, horny surface. May change color dramatically from thrombosis. Solitary lesion; most on the lower extremities.

Venous lake: Dark red papule, compressed with fingertips. Usually in older patients.

Dermatofibroma: Asymptomatic, firm papule, sharply circumscribed. May result from minor trauma. Can be dark brown to black. Usually less than 1 cm in diameter.

Seborrheic keratosis: Common growth in middle-aged and elderly patients. Frequently occurs on face and trunk. "Stuck-on" appearance. Color ranges from brown to black.

Pigmented basal cell carcinoma: Pearly appearance with dark brown pigmentation. More frequent in Spanish or Asian patients.

TABLE 8 ABCDE GUIDELINES FOR DIAGNOSIS OF MALIGNANT MELANOMA

Asymmetry: Benign nevi are symmetric, melanomas tend to have pronounced asymmetry
Border: Benign nevi have smooth borders, melanomas have notched, irregular outlines
Color: Benign nevi usually are at one color, melanomas usually have a variegated color
Diameter: Benign nevi are usually smaller than 6 mm in diameter
Elevation: Malignant melanoma is almost always elevated above the skin surface

TABLE 9 COMMON DISTANT SITES OF METASTATIC MELANOMA

Site	Incidence
Skin and lymph nodes	42%–59%
Lungs	18%–36%
Liver	14%–20%
Brain	12%–20%
Bones	11%–17%
Intestines	1%–7%

Classification of Melanoma

It has become clear that different melanoma tumors vary in their clinical and growth characteristics. Based on this, melanomas have been classified into four somewhat arbitrary subtypes: superficial spreading melanoma, nodular melanoma, lentigo maligna melanoma, and acral lentiginous melanoma.

Each subtype presents with unique clinical characteristics and prognoses (Figs. 13–20). Lentigo maligna, superficial spreading melanoma (Figs. 21–23), and acral lentiginous melanoma initially spread horizontally and only subsequently invade vertically. In fact, the lentigo maligna variant spreads horizontally for years before invading into the deeper layers of the skin. This is the reason for the excellent prognosis associated with this subtype. In contrast, the nodular subtype has virtually no horizontal growth phase and penetrates into the deeper layers of the skin from the start. It is thereby associated with a much worse prognosis.

Superficial spreading melanoma is the most common histologic variant among whites, and overall accounts for approximately 70% of the cases. It most frequently occurs in younger patients, usually in their fourth to fifth decade of life. It most commonly occurs on the trunk in men and legs in women.

Nodular melanoma usually arises in the fifth to sixth decade of life and is associated with a poor prognosis. It does not have a horizontal growth phase and is associated with nodules of invasive tumor. It occurs more commonly in men and most commonly on the trunk and extremities.

Lentigo maligna melanoma comprises approximately 4% to 10% of melanomas and usually occurs on the face of an elderly person. While still in its horizontal growth phase, it is called lentigo maligna, and appears as a flat, pigmented lesion that gradually enlarges over time. It has irregular borders and the colors in the lesion are variegated. If allowed to proceed, the pigmented lesion thickens as it invades into the dermis. It is then known as lentigo maligna melanoma.

Acral lentiginous melanoma comprises approximately 10% of all melanomas in whites but approximately 50% of all melanomas in blacks, Asians, and Hispanics. Most lesions occur underneath the nails (subungual melanoma) and on the plantar aspect of the feet.

Subungual melanoma should be differentiated from melanonychia striata, a dark streak that runs longitudinally in the nail plate. Melanonychia striata is benign and results from increased melanin deposition in the nail plate. Table 10 lists clues that favor the diagnosis of melanoma (malignant) over melanonychia striata (benign). The latter occurs more commonly in darkly pigmented people and is unusual in whites. A higher level of suspicion should be directed toward a single streak in a patient whose other nails are completely unaffected. Multiple pigmented streaks or a solitary streak in a black person is more likely to be benign. An enlarging or changing streak also deserves careful attention. The spread of pigmentation beyond the nail into the proximal or lateral nail folds also indicates a greater likelihood for melanoma. After clinical examination, if there is still any doubt about the diagnosis, a biopsy should be performed. Subungual melanomas are associated with a poor prognosis, with 5-year survival rates in the range of 30% to 40%.

(Text continues on page 122)

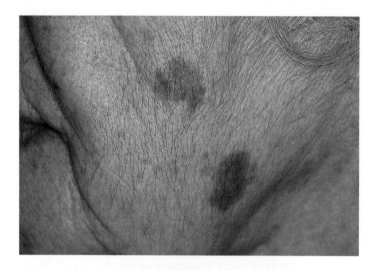

Figure 13
Solar lentigo. This sun-induced tan macule is entirely benign.

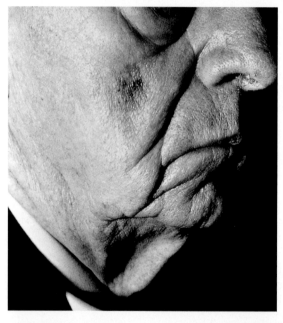

Figure 14
Lentigo maligna, a premalignant melanocytic neoplasm. Note the variegation in color.

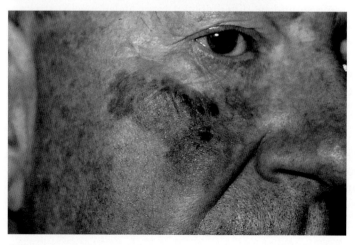

Figure 15
Lentigo maligna. Because of the large size of the lesion, an incisional biopsy of the darker areas should be carried out to establish the diagnosis.

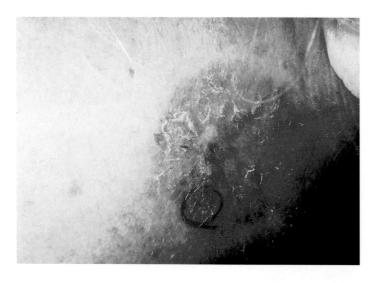

Figure 16
Lentigo maligna. A punch biopsy of the darker-pigmented area established the diagnosis.

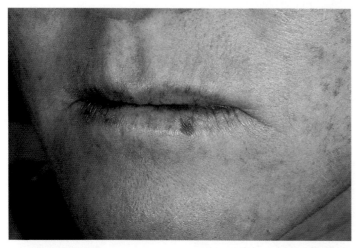

Figure 17
Lentigo on the lower lip. This is a benign lesion.

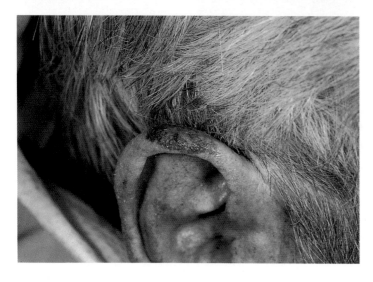

Figure 18
Lentigo maligna, helical rim.

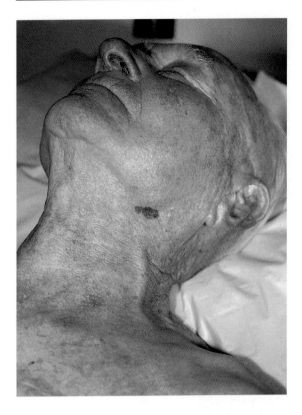

Figure 19

Lentigo maligna. The tumor remains in the horizontal growth phase for a prolonged period, but if left untreated, it may eventually progress to lentigo maligna melanoma and spread.

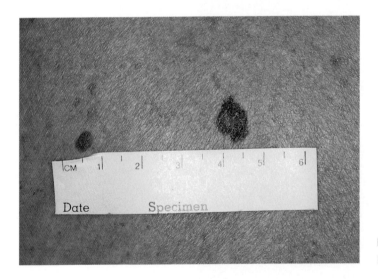

Figure 20

Lentigo maligna, back.

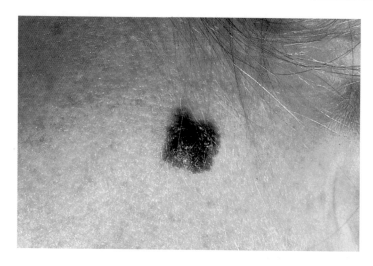

Figure 21

Superficial spreading melanoma. Variegation of color and irregularity of borders is evident.

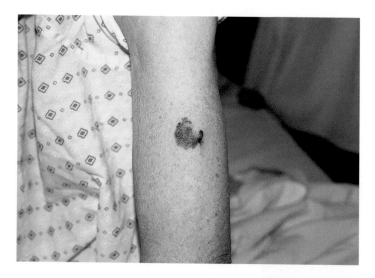

Figure 22

Superficial spreading melanoma. This is the most common histologic variant of melanoma.

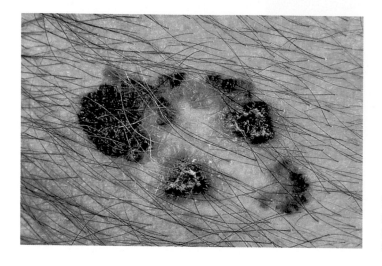

Figure 23

Superficial spreading melanoma. The irregular appearance should prompt a biopsy.

**TABLE 10 CLUES THAT FAVOR THE DIAGNOSIS
OF MELANOMA (MALIGNANT) OVER MELANONYCHIA
STRIATA (BENIGN)**

Only a single digit is involved
Pigmentation develops in a previously normal nail
Pigmentation suddenly becomes darker or wider
Positive personal history or family history of melanoma
Blurred lateral borders
Extension of pigment to surrounding skin

Pathology

Histopathologically, malignant melanoma (Figs. 24–26) presents as a proliferation of atypical malignant melanocytes spreading throughout the epidermis as either single cells or in groups. The tumor always originates at the dermal–epidermal junction. The melanoma cells spread both downward into the underlying dermis as well as extending upward into the overlying epidermis. The melanoma cells usually have a prominent and atypical-appearing nucleus. In the dermis, the tumor cells show great variation in size and shape. Depending on the host, there may be a small or large number of inflammatory cells present around the tumor. Table 11 lists other prognostic features that need to be considered.

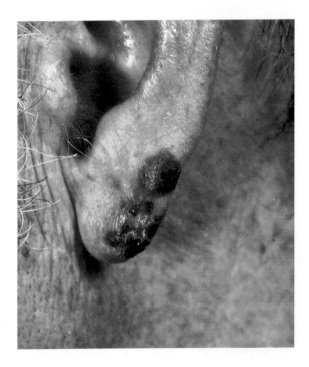

Figure 24

Malignant melanoma, left earlobe. Note the asymmetry, border irregularity, color variegation, and large diameter of the lesion.

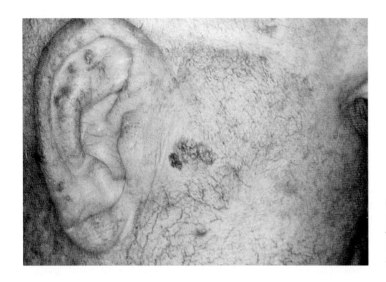

Figure 25

Lentigo maligna melanoma on the right preauricle with satellite metastatic lesions on the ear.

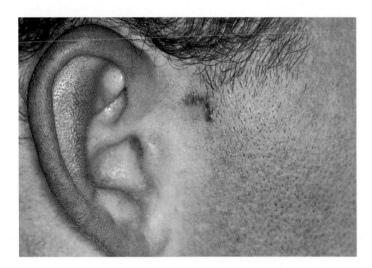

Figure 26

Malignant melanoma. This 34-year-old patient complained of this new-onset pigmented lesion. Biopsy of the lesion showed a Clark level II malignant melanoma.

TABLE 11 OTHER PROGNOSTIC FEATURES THAT NEED TO BE CONSIDERED IN MELANOMA

Extremity lesions in general have better prognosis than lesions on the trunk.

Survival rates are worse for ulcerated melanomas compared with nonulcerated melanomas when matched for thickness and stage of disease.

Women have a better prognosis than men when matched for tumor thickness.

On histopathologic evaluation, the presence of lymphocytic infiltrate at base of the lesion and infiltrating the tumor is associated with a better prognosis.

Patients younger than 50 years of age have a better prognosis than patients older than 50.

Diagnosis

It is imperative that all suspect pigmented lesions be sampled for biopsy, because clinical inspection alone is not enough to exclude a diagnosis of melanoma (Table 12). Many skin lesions may clinically resemble malignant melanoma (see Table 7). With clinical experience, the physician becomes better able to differentiate between benign and malignant lesions. In fact, studies have shown that as many as one third of biopsy-proven melanomas were misdiagnosed before biopsy. Once a lesion has enough atypical features to render it suspect for malignancy, the threshold for biopsy should be low. The importance of early biopsy of suspect lesions cannot be overemphasized. Figures 9 through 13 depict some of the more common entities that may be mistaken for melanoma.

Several methods may be used for biopsy of suspected melanoma lesions, including excisional, incisional, and punch biopsy. Excisional biopsy is preferred because it allows the pathologist to evaluate the entire specimen and thus make a more accurate diagnosis. The excision is carried out with 2-mm margins around the tumor and should include full-thickness skin along with subcutaneous fat. An important point is to orient the excision such that the long axis is in the direction of lymph flow. After the excision, the specimen should be oriented using a single suture before submission in formalin for histopathologic evaluation. Punch biopsy may be used in excisional surgery of small lesions. In these cases, a punch biopsy instrument should be selected that is 1 to 2 mm greater in diameter than the lesion. A punch instrument may also be used for incisional biopsy (removal of only a portion of the lesion). An incisional biopsy should be used only for those lesions that are either large (>2 cm) or located on sensitive anatomic areas. If an incisional punch biopsy is used, the most raised site or the darkest area of the lesion should be sampled.

Shave biopsy for lesions suspect for melanoma is not recommended because the pathologist may not be able to make an optimal diagnosis. In addition, tumor thickness cannot be measured, and thus prognostic information cannot be provided. This emphasizes the importance of obtaining a specimen of full thickness for the accurate determination of prognosis and treatment plans.

If histopathologic evaluation confirms the diagnosis of melanoma, then a second stage of surgical excision must be carried out. The excision should be extended to the level of the fascia, with the margins of the excision directly dependent on the thickness of the tumor.

TABLE 12 GUIDELINES FOR BIOPSY OF PIGMENTED LESIONS

Biopsy Indicated
    Change in preexisting nevus: itching, bleeding, change in size or color
    Pigmented lesion satisfying all of the ABCDE criteria

Consider Biopsy
    De novo pigmented lesion satisfying any combination of the ABCDE criteria

TABLE 13 CLARK'S LEVELS OF INVASION

Level I	All tumor cells above basement membrane; also termed *in situ* melanoma
Level II	Tumor cells have broken through basement membrane and extend into papillary dermis, but have not entered reticular dermis
Level III	Tumor cells have invaded ill-defined interface between papillar and reticular dermis
Level IV	Neoplastic cells are seen between collagen bundles of reticular dermis
Level V	Neoplastic cells have invaded subcutaneous tissue

Staging/Prognosis

Malignant melanoma is staged according to the Breslow classification, which uses the vertical thickness of the tumor (measured from the top of the granular layer to the deepest point [see Fig. 26] of tumor penetration), or Clark's classification, which examines the anatomic level of invasion (Table 13). The Breslow classification of tumor thickness has been shown to be more accurate in indicating the prognosis associated with the tumor. However, in areas with thin skin, such as the eyelid or the ear, the Clark level of invasion is an important prognostic tool.

Although the depth of penetration of the tumor is the most important prognostic variable, other factors such as age and sex of the patient, the anatomic location, and histologic evaluation are all important variables that should be considered (Figs. 27–66).

The American Joint Commission on Cancer has created the most current and widely used staging system, based on the TNM (**t**umor, **n**odes, **m**etastasis) classification (Table 14). Table 15 describes recurrence in patients with stage I melanoma. Based on the stage of the disease, careful recommendations for follow-up have been set forth.

(Text continues on page 142)

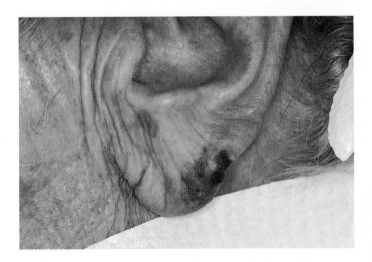

Figure 27

Malignant melanoma, left earlobe. Despite aggressive intervention, the patient later died of metastatic disease.

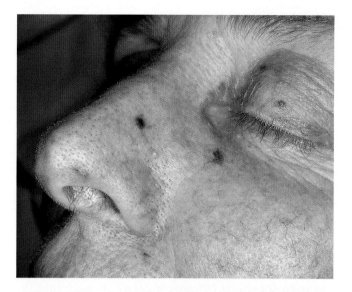

Figure 28
Malignant melanoma. Although the characteristic features of melanoma are missing, the history of recent onset and the dark hue of the lesion prompted a biopsy that confirmed the diagnosis.

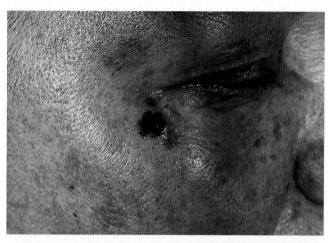

Figure 29
Malignant melanoma.

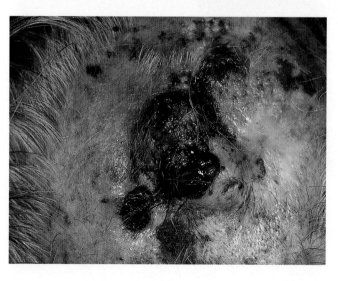

Figure 30
Metastatic malignant melanoma.

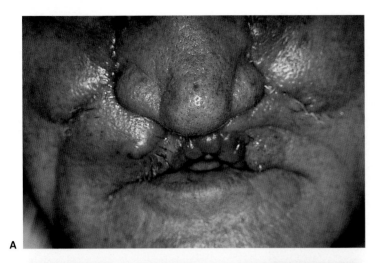

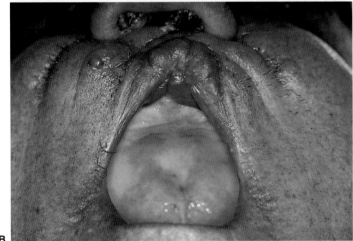

Figure 31

(A,B) Recurrent malignant melanoma, upper lip. The tumor recurred in its original location despite initial aggressive intervention.

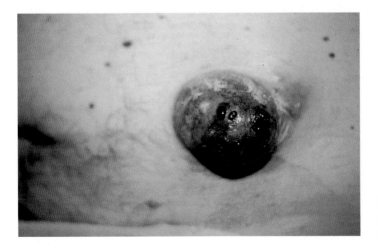

Figure 32

Nodular malignant melanoma, advanced.

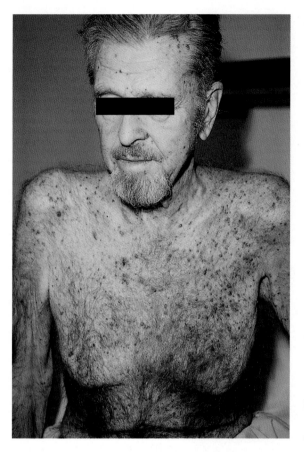

Figure 33

Metastatic malignant melanoma. This man died shortly after the photograph was taken.

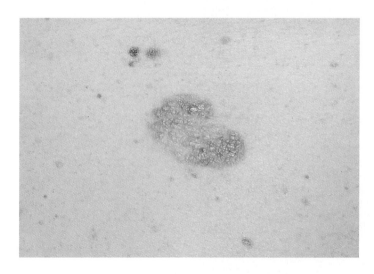

Figure 34

Amelanotic malignant melanoma. Note the absence of pigment. Fortunately, this entity is relatively rare.

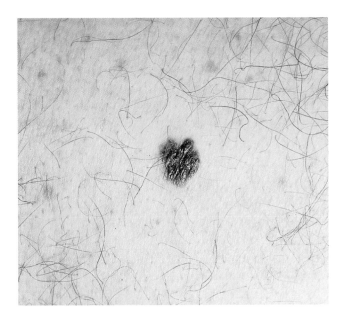

Figure 35
Malignant melanoma. The variegation in color is rather prominent.

Figure 36
Nodular malignant melanoma. The characteristic features rendering the lesion suspect for melanoma are absent.

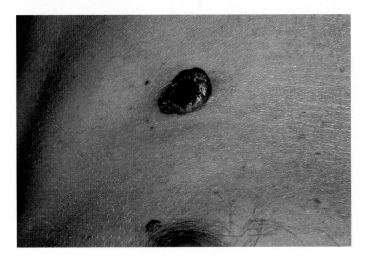

Figure 37
Nodular malignant melanoma.

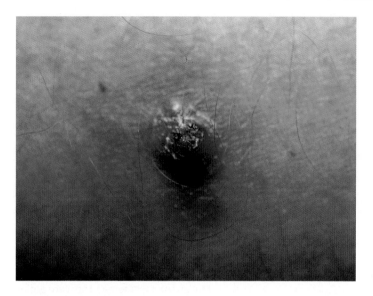

Figure 38

Malignant melanoma. Friable tumor on the trunk. Biopsy confirmed the diagnosis.

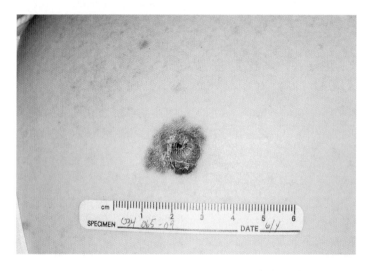

Figure 39

Malignant melanoma. Biopsy indicated a tumor thickness of 3.2 mm.

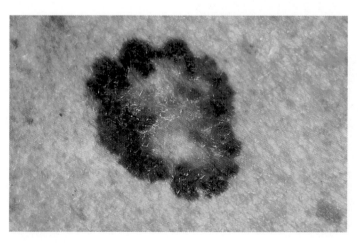

Figure 40

Malignant melanoma. Annular pigmentation with central clearing is seen in this particular tumor.

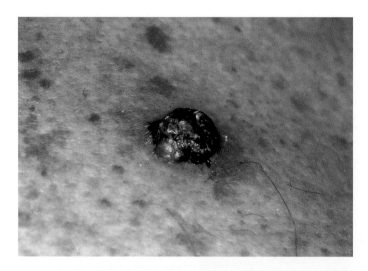

Figure 41
Note the strong inflammatory response to the tumor.

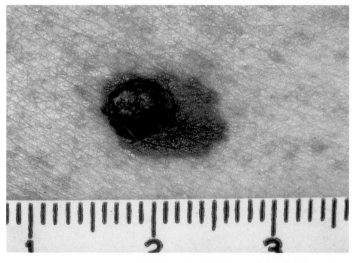

Figure 42
Malignant melanoma. Note the black nodular component.

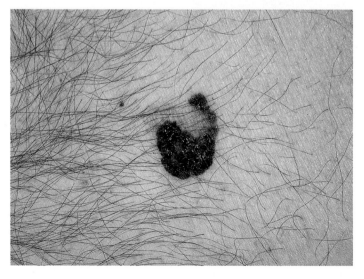

Figure 43
Nodular malignant melanoma on the abdomen.

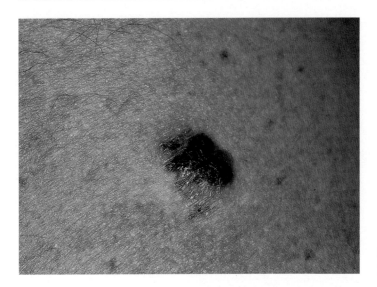

Figure 44
Malignant melanoma.

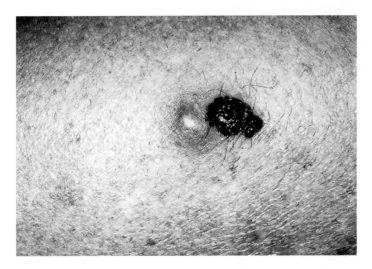

Figure 45
Malignant melanoma. Note the amelanotic portion of the tumor.

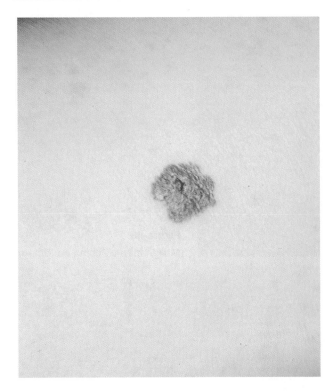

Figure 46

Malignant melanoma. The legs are the most common site in women.

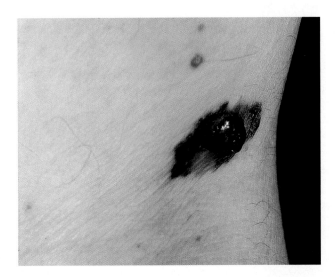

Figure 47

Malignant melanoma. As with most melanomas, this lesion arose on normal skin.

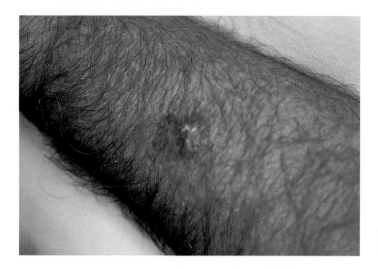

Figure 48
Malignant melanoma on the arm.

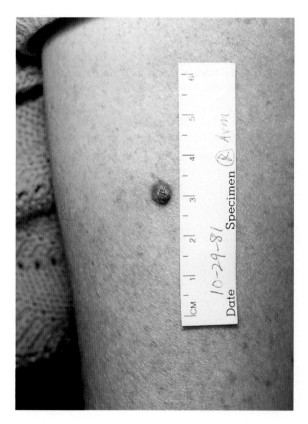

Figure 49
Nodular malignant melanoma. This tumor penetrates deep in a short period of time. Note the asymmetric appearance of the lesion.

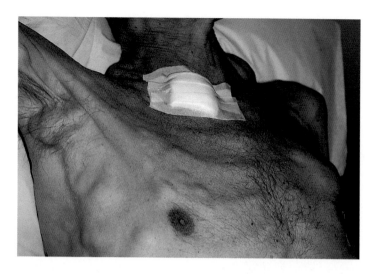

Figure 50

Metastatic malignant melanoma. The multiple subcutaneous tumors all represent metastatic disease.

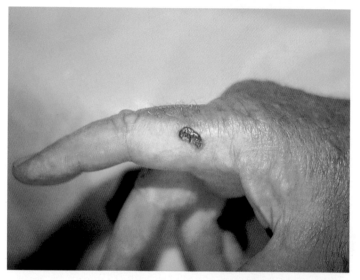

Figure 51

Malignant melanoma. This tumor could easily be confused with a vascular tumor.

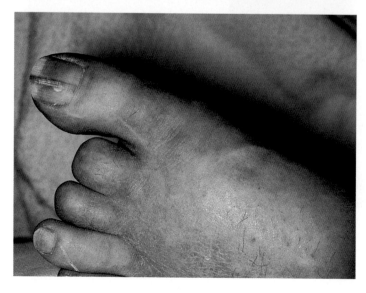

Figure 52

Subungual malignant melanoma. This patient in her mid-40s presented with a history of a recent-onset pigmented band on her large toenail. Biopsy of the nail plate revealed a malignant process.

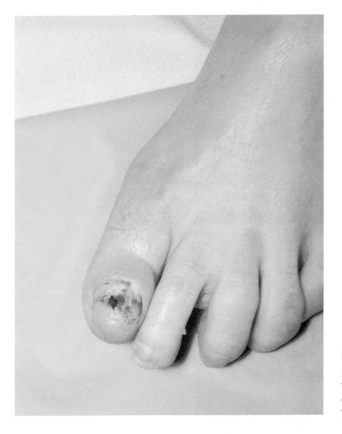

Figure 53

Subungual malignant melanoma. This tumor was ignored by the patient and eventually caused the destruction of the nail plate.

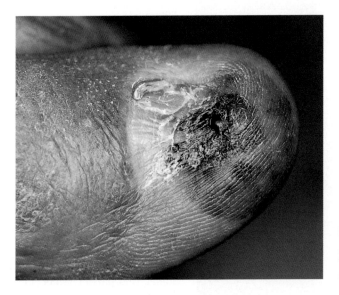

Figure 54

Acral lentiginous melanoma. Note that the pigment extends into the surrounding skin.

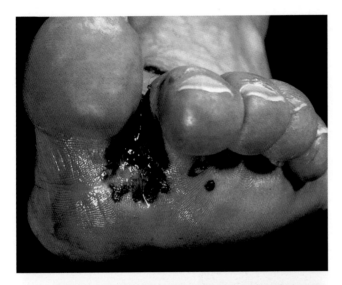

Figure 55
Acral lentiginous melanoma. This form of melanoma occurs more commonly in blacks, Asians, and Hispanics.

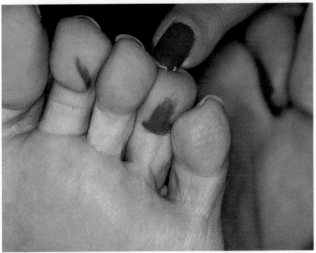

Figure 56
Acral lentiginous melanoma. Despite aggressive intervention, including amputation and adjuvant therapy, the patient eventually died of metastases.

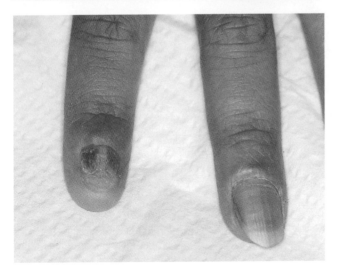

Figure 57
Acral lentiginous melanoma in a young Hispanic woman.

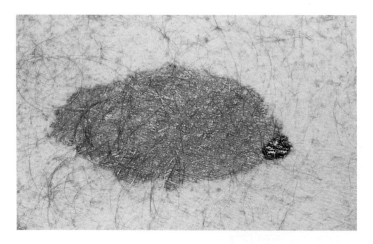

Figure 58
Malignant melanoma arising in a congenital nevus.

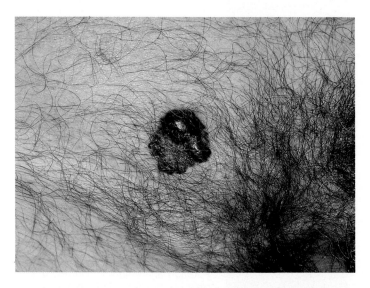

Figure 59
Pigmented basal cell carcinoma. The clinical appearance may lead the physician to arrive immediately at the diagnosis of melanoma. Fortunately, a shave biopsy showed otherwise.

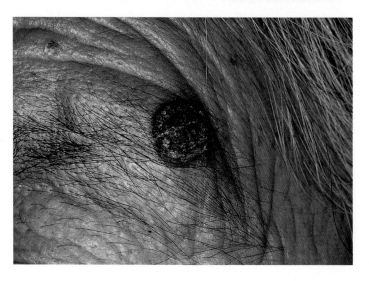

Figure 60
Seborrheic keratosis. This is a completely benign tumor without any sequelae.

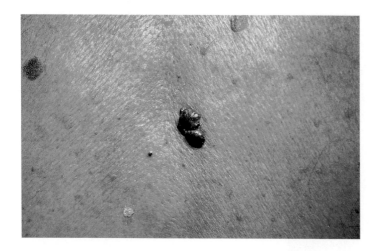

Figure 61

Malignant melanoma on the back. This tumor was identified during a routine screening; the patient was completely unaware of its presence.

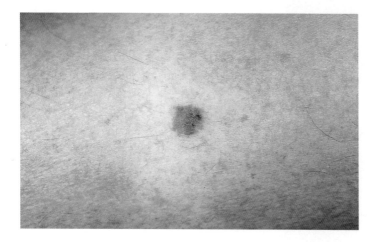

Figure 62

Seborrheic keratosis. An unusual appearance, but this tumor can sometimes mimic a melanoma.

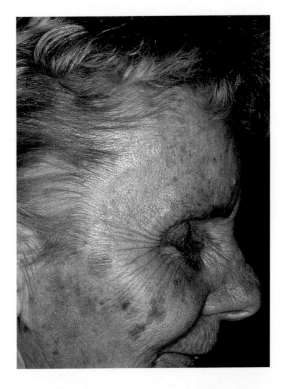

Figure 63
Multiple solar lentigos due to extensive sun damage.

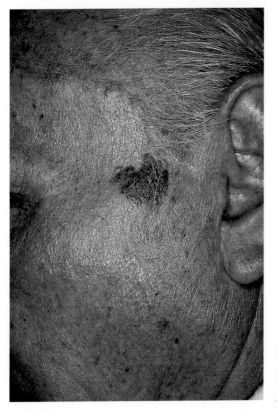

Figure 64
Seborrheic keratosis. The verrucous appearance of this lesion may be a clue to its benignity. Regardless, pathologic documentation is required.

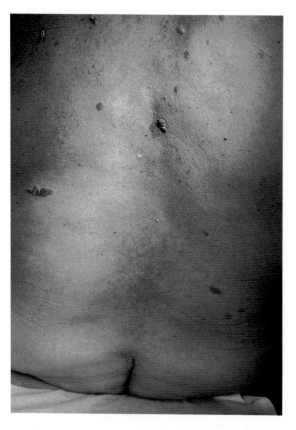

Figure 65

Malignant melanoma on the central back amid multiple seborrheic keratosis.

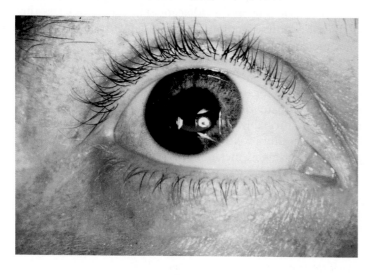

Figure 66

Malignant melanoma. This tumor had extended onto the conjunctiva. The prognosis for such tumors is relatively poor.

TABLE 14 STAGING OF CUTANEOUS MELANOMA

Stage I	Localized disease
Stage II	Regional lymph node involvement
Stage III	Distant metastatic disease

TABLE 15 RECURRENCE IN PATIENTS WITH STAGE I MELANOMA

Tumor Thickness (mm)	5-Year Survival Rate (%)	Recurrence
<0.76	96	1%/y × 3–5 y
0.76–1.49	87	5%/y × 3–5 y
1.50–2.49	75	12%–19%/y × 1st 2 y
		5%/y × next 3 y
2.50–3.99	66	12%–19%/y × 1st 2 y
		5%/y × next 3 y
> 4.00	47	30%/y × 1st y
		12%/y × next 3 y

Treatment

The width of the surgical margin for excision of primary melanoma of the skin has been the object of much debate among cutaneous surgeons for many years. A wide local excision with 5-cm margins was widely advocated early in the 20th century. Although disfiguring, the treatment was deemed justified because of its ability to remove "microscopic satellites" in the adjacent skin. Early in the 1970s, after Clark and Breslow provided prognostic data correlating tumor thickness to survival rate, a trend began toward more conservative approaches to the management and treatment of primary cutaneous melanoma. Breslow showed that in melanomas less than 0.76 mm in thickness, the width of the resection margin had no effect on the rate of local recurrence or metastasis. Another large study showed no microscopic satellites of tumor cells in the adjacent skin for lesions less than 0.75 mm in thickness. Based on these findings, a conservative resection margin was proposed for thinner melanomas (Tables 16–18).

However, microscopic satellites of tumor cells in the surrounding skin were found to increase dramatically as the thickness of the lesion increased. Wider resection margins were thus proposed for these thicker tumors. Currently, a 2- to 3-cm margin has been deemed adequate for melanomas greater than 1 mm in thickness. Wider surgical margins are probably not of significant clinical value even for thicker melanomas. Table 19 describes follow-up recommendations according to tumor thickness for patients with stage I melanomas.

**TABLE 16 FIVE-YEAR SURVIVAL RATES
FOR CLINICAL STAGE I MELANOMA
ACCORDING TO BRESLOW THICKNESS**

Tumor Thickness (mm)	Survival (%)
<0.76	96
0.76–1.49	87
1.50–2.49	75
2.50–3.99	66
>4	47

**TABLE 17 FIVE-YEAR SURVIVAL RATES
FOR CLINICAL STAGE I MELANOMA
ACCORDING TO CLARK'S LEVEL OF INVASION**

Clark's Level	Survival (%)
II	85–100
III	73–88
IV	43–66
V	15–33

**TABLE 18 RECOMMENDED SURGICAL
MARGINS BASED ON TUMOR THICKNESS**

Tumor Thickness	Margins (cm)
Melanoma-*in-situ*	0.5
<1 mm	1
>1 mm	2–3

Surgical margins greater than 2 to 3 cm are probably not of significant clinical value even for thicker melanomas.

**TABLE 19 FOLLOW-UP RECOMMENDATIONS ACCORDING TO TUMOR THICKNESS FOR PATIENTS
WITH STAGE I MELANOMA**

Lesions <0.76 mm in thickness
    Screening: No studies
    Follow-up: Yearly for life
    Laboratory evaluation: Only to confirm clinical suspicion

Lesions 0.76–1.50 mm in thickness
    Screening: Chest radiograph
    Follow-up: Chest radiograph yearly for 5 years
    History and physical: Every 6 months for 3 years; every year thereafter

Lesions >1.50 mm in thickness
    Screening: Chest CT scan plus serum LDH; if LDH elevated, then abdominal CT scan
    Follow-up, first and second years
        1.51–3 mm thick
        Chest radiograph every year
        Physician visit every 3 months
        >3 mm thick
        Chest radiograph every 6 months first year
        Every year thereafter
        Physician visit every 3 months
        LDH at end of second year
    Follow-up, third and fourth years
        Chest radiograph every year
        Physician visit every 6 months
    Follow-up, fifth year and beyond
        Physician visit every year
        Laboratory evaluation only to confirm clinical suspicion

CT, computed tomography; LDH, lactate dehydrogenase.

From Rogers GS. Advances in diagnostic technique. *J Dermatol Surg Oncol* 1989; 15:605–607.
With permission.

Mohs Micrographic Surgery

Although firmly established as the treatment of choice for basal cell carcinoma and squamous cell carcinomas in certain anatomic areas, Mohs surgery remains a controversial technique when used in the treatment of melanoma. The controversy has centered around the difficulty encountered in the identification of melanoma cells on frozen section. The advantage of this technique is that 100% of the surgical margin—the entire periphery and undersurface of the specimen—is examined for subclinical extensions of tumor while sparing normal tissue. Using Mohs surgery, the visible tumor is excised with a 6-mm surgical margin, extending to the subcutaneous fat. A 2-mm surgical margin is then taken around the wound for evaluation by frozen-section analysis.

Elective Regional Lymph Node Dissection

Elective lymphadenectomy for malignant melanoma continues to be an extremely controversial topic. The hypothesis has been set forth that melanoma spreads sequentially from the primary lesion to the regional lymph nodes before distant metastasis. Under this theory, the lymph node acts as a biologic filter, stopping melanoma from metastasizing. The aim of elective lymphadenectomy is to circumvent the distant spread of melanoma in those patients who have had a metastasis to a regional lymph node. Large-scale, prospective, randomized studies have not shown any therapeutic benefit associated with elective lymph node dissection.

Sentinel node evaluation is a newer technique in which a dye is used to help determine the pattern of lymph node drainage from the tumor. On establishing the route of drainage, the surgical oncologist samples this area to determine whether the tumor has spread to the regional lymph nodes. If pathologic study reveals tumor, surgical lymphadenectomy of the area is undertaken. However, the value of this technique remains unclear.

In December 1995, adjuvant therapy with α-interferon was approved for certain advanced melanomas. Gene transfer studies using tumor-infiltrating lymphocytes combined with interleukin-2 are currently underway. Further discussion of this and other adjuvant treatment modalities is beyond the scope of this book.

Table 20 lists important signs that may provide a clue to the diagnosis of melanoma. Different clinical signs may present based on the pattern in which a melanoma has metastasized.

TABLE 20 IMPORTANT POINTS IN THE HISTORY IN EVALUATING PATIENTS WITH MELANOMA FOR METASTATIC DISEASE

Skin: New or changing lesion
Brain: Persisting headache, specific motor or sensory deficits
Bone: Localized pain
Gastrointestinal tract: Hematemesis, melena, obstruction, pain
Kidneys: Hematuria
Liver: Weight loss, right upper quadrant abdominal pain
Lungs: Dyspnea, cough, hemoptysis

Suggested Readings

Blois MS, Sagebiel RW, Abarbanel RM, Caldwell TM, Tuttle MS. Malignant melanoma of the skin: 1. the association of tumor depth and type, and patient sex, age, and site with survival. *Cancer* 1983;52:1330–1341.

Briele HA, Beattie CW, Ronanana SG, et al. Late recurrence of cutaneous melanoma. *Arch Surg* 1983;118:800–803.

Coleman WP III, David RS, Reed RJ, et al. Treatment of lentigo maligna and lentigo maligna melanoma. *Journal of Dermatologic and Surgical Oncology* 1980;6:476–479.

Day CL Jr, Mihm MC Jr, Sober AJ, et al. Narrower margins for clinical stage I melanoma patients. *N Engl J Med* 1982;306:479–481.

Day CL Jr, Mihm MC Jr, Sober AJ, et al. Prognostic factors for melanoma patients with lesions 0.76 mm–1.69 mm in thickness: an appraisal of "thin" level IV lesions. *Ann Surg* 1982;195:30–34.

Ho VC, Sober AJ. Therapy for cutaneous melanoma: an update. *J Am Acad Dermatol* 1990;22:159–176.

Koh HK, Sober AJ, Harmon DC, Lew RA, Carey RW. Adjuvant therapy of cutaneous malignant melanoma: a critical review. *Med Pediatr Oncol* 1985;13:244–266.

Kopf AW, Mintzis M, Bart RS. Diagnostic accuracy in malignant melanoma. *Arch Dermatol* 1975;111:1291–1292.

Kopf AW, Hellman LJ, Rogers GS, et al. Familial malignant melanoma. *JAMA* 1986;256:1915–1919.

Longstreth J. Cutaneous malignant melanoma and ultraviolet radiation: a review. *Cancer Metastasis Rev* 1988;7:321–333.

Rao BN, Hayes FA, Pratt CB, et al. Malignant melanoma in children: its management and prognosis. *J Pediatr Surg* 1990;25:198–203.

Thorn M, Adami HO, Bergstrom R, Ringburg U, Krusemo UB. Trends in survival from malignant melanoma: remarkable improvement in 23 years. *J Natl Cancer Inst* 1989;81:611–617.

Veronesi U, Cascinelli N, Adamus J, et al. Thin stage I primary cutaneous malignant melanoma. *N Engl J Med* 1988;318:1159–1162.

White MJ, Polk AC. Therapy of primary cutaneous melanomas. *Med Clin North Am* 1986;70:71–87.

CHAPTER 6

SEBACEOUS CARCINOMA

Clinical Features

Sebaceous carcinoma is another rare malignant tumor of the skin (Fig. 1). It is a solitary, firm, flesh-colored to yellow papule that occurs most commonly on the upper eyelid in the sixth to eighth decade of life. It does occasionally present at other cutaneous sites on the face and scalp. The tumors vary in their growth pattern (Fig. 2); some grow rapidly with early invasion, whereas others evolve very slowly. Sebaceous carcinoma occurs more commonly in Asians and those with a history of previous radiation therapy. Clinically, it may mimic a chalazion or a chronic conjunctivitis (Table 1). Despite its innocent appearance, it is an aggressive tumor and has a high rate of local recurrence and distant metastasis (Table 2). Organs most commonly affected are the regional nodes, lung, liver, and brain.

Sebaceous carcinoma may occur less commonly on nonocular tissue. Although initially thought to be less aggressive than its periocular counterparts, it is now known that these tumors also have a high rate of recurrence and metastasis.

Sebaceous carcinomas arise in meibomian glands and occasionally from the glands of Zeis in the periocular tissue. The sebaceous glands associated with the fine lanugo hairs of the face give rise to the nonocular tumors.

Pathogenesis

The etiology of sebaceous carcinoma is unknown. Ultraviolet light as well as irradiation are likely contributing factors.

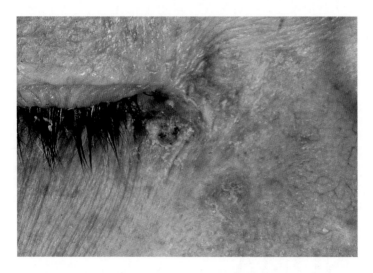

Figure 1

Sebaceous carcinoma. This yellowish papule arose in the periocular region of an elderly woman.

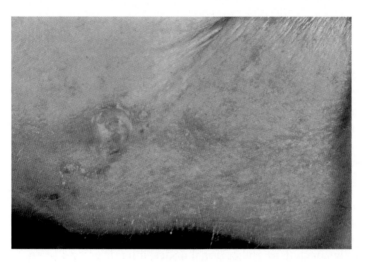

Figure 2

Sebaceous carcinoma. It has an innocent appearance, but is a highly aggressive tumor.

TABLE 1 CLINICAL CHARACTERISTICS OF SEBACEOUS CARCINOMA

Average age: 57 years
Sex predilection: Woman slightly outnumber men
Anatomic site: Most commonly on the upper eyelids
Prognosis: High rate of recurrence and metastasis

TABLE 2 RISK OF RECURRENCE AND METASTASIS FOR SEBACEOUS CARCINOMAS IN PERIOCULAR AND NONOCULAR TISSUE

	Recurrence Rate (%)	Metastatic Rate (%)
Periocular tissue	33	30
Nonocular tissue	34	32

Histopathology

A multilobular configuration of basophilic cells containing nests of vacuolated cells is present deep in the dermis. The individual cells have a foamy, vacuolated cytoplasm with round, centrally placed nuclei. Light microscopy reveals pleomorphic cells with bizarre nuclei and a high mitotic index. Signs of local tissue invasion may be present. Immunohistochemistry shows strong epithelial membrane antigen expression.

Diagnosis

The tumor is rarely diagnosed clinically and may be mistaken for a variety of other entities, including chalazion, blepharoconjunctivitis, sebaceous adenoma, epithelioma, basal cell carcinoma, and squamous cell carcinoma. A chalazion often appears as an inflamed papule that rapidly enlarges along the ciliary margin of the eye. Sebaceous carcinoma should also be differentiated from sebaceous epithelioma and sebaceous adenoma, which may have a similar appearance clinically. Histopathologically, it is much less pleomorphic and has a more regular lobular architecture. A low threshold should exist for the biopsy of suspect lesions to establish an accurate diagnosis.

On making the diagnosis of sebaceous carcinoma, a careful work-up is required to rule out distant metastasis (Table 3). Sebaceous carcinoma has also been associated with internal, especially gastrointestinal malignancies (Muir-Torre syndrome).

Treatment

Because of its aggressive nature and high rate of recurrence, wide surgical excision of the tumor with orbital exenteration is a must. Mohs micrographic surgery has been used successfully to attain better margin control while conserving tissue. Various reports to date have shown outstanding results.

Radiation therapy has been used to treat sebaceous carcinoma both as a primary modality and as adjuvant therapy. The disadvantage of this technique lies in the inability to ensure tumor-free margins subsequent to treatment.

Extension of the tumor into the orbit significantly worsens the prognosis. For these cases, orbital exenteration needs to be performed.

TABLE 3 MOST COMMON SITES OF DISTANT METASTASIS FOR SEBACEOUS CARCINOMA

Regional nodes
Lung
Liver
Brain

Prognosis

Because of its aggressive nature, a careful follow-up of patients with sebaceous carcinoma is indicated. There is a high incidence of metastases to the regional lymph nodes at the time of diagnosis. If treated aggressively with lymph node dissection, there appears to be a 50% 5-year survival rate.

Suggested Readings

Beach A, Seerance AO. Sebaceous gland carcinoma. *Ann Surg* 1942;115:258.

Doxanas MT, Green WR. Sebaceous gland carcinoma: review of 40 cases. *Arch Ophthalmol* 1984;102:245–249.

Folberg R, Whitaker DC, Tse DT, Nerad JA. Recurrent and residual sebaceous carcinoma after Mohs excision of the primary lesion. *Am J Ophthalmol* 1987;103:817–823.

King DT, Hirose FM, Gurevitch AW. Sebaceous carcinoma of the skin with visceral metastases. *Arch Dermatol* 1979;115:862–863.

Miller RE, White JJ. Sebaceous gland carcinoma. *Am J Surg* 1981;114:958–961.

Nunery WR, Welsh MG, MCord CD. Recurrence of sebaceous carcinoma of the eyelid after radiation therapy. *Am J Ophthalmol* 1983;96:10–15.

Rao NA, Hidayat AA, McLean IW, Zimmerman LE. Sebaceous carcinomas of the ocular adnexa: a clinicopathologic study of 104 cases, with five-year follow-up data. *Hum Pathol* 1982;13:113–122.

Ratz JL, Lun-Duong S, Kulwin DR. Sebaceous carcinoma of the eyelid treated with Mohs surgery. *J Am Acad Dermatol* 1986;14:668–673.

Rothenberg J, Lambert WC, Vail JT, et al. The Muir-Torre syndrome: the significance of a solitary sebaceous tumor. *J Am Acad Dermatol* 1990;23:638–640.

Schlernitzauer DA, Font RL. Sebaceous gland carcinoma of the eyelid. *Arch Ophthalmol* 1976;94:1523–1525.

Wagoner MD, Beyer CK, Gonder JR, et al. Common presentations of sebaceous gland carcinoma of the eyelid. *Ophthalmology* 1982;14:159–163.

CHAPTER 7

MERKEL CELL CARCINOMA

Merkel cell carcinoma is a rare, highly aggressive, relatively undifferentiated malignant tumor of the skin that shows a propensity for sun-damaged skin. The tumor has features of both neural and epithelial differentiation. It is also known as "neuroendocrine carcinoma of the skin." The tumor is often found in association with epithelial nerve endings. Ultrastructural studies show distinct neurosecretory granules in the cytoplasm of the Merkel cells.

Merkel cells are believed to function as receptors for mechanical stimuli. Animal studies have shown that Merkel cells act as slowly adapting mechanoreceptors that fire with high frequency on detection of even slight mechanical movement. On sensing movement, Merkel cells cause the attached dermal nerve fibers to transduce an electric signal, and thereby act as receptors capable of transducing physical to chemical activity.

Clinical Features

Merkel cell carcinoma typically presents as a solitary, firm, red to violaceous, dome-shaped nodule with occasional overlying telangiectases and surrounding erythema (Table 1 and Fig. 1). It usually measures less than 2 cm in diameter and slowly increases in size. It almost always occurs as a single lesion, although multiple tumors have been described. Ulceration and bleeding may be associated features.

Merkel cell carcinoma most commonly occurs in people older than 65 years of age, although patients as young as 7 years of age have been afflicted. The sex distribution is approximately equal. Whites are the most commonly affected, although rare cases have been reported in blacks. The face and neck are the most common locations for the tumor (>50%), followed by the upper extremities

TABLE 1 CLINICAL FEATURES OF MERKEL CELL CARCINOMA AT PRESENTATION

Age	
Average	68 years
Range	15–97 years
Sex	
48% male, 52% female	
Primary anatomic site	
Head and neck	49%
Upper extremities	16%
Lower extremities	20%
Trunk	4%
Multiple	1.5%

From Hitchcock CL, Bland KI, Laney RG, et al. Neuroendocrine (Merkel cell) carcinoma of the skin: its natural history, diagnosis, and treatment. *Ann Surg* 1988;207: 201–207, with permission.

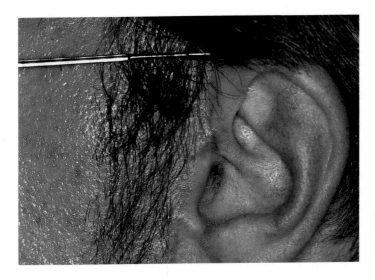

Figure 1

Merkel cell carcinoma: a solitary, firm, dome-shaped nodule. Its nonspecific appearance may lead to a mistaken diagnosis.

TABLE 2 HISTOLOGIC DIFFERENTIAL DIAGNOSIS OF MERKEL CELL CARCINOMA

Cutaneous lymphoma
Malignant melanoma
Sweat gland carcinoma
Metastatic small cell lung carcinoma
Metastatic neuroblastoma
Squamous cell carcinoma
Cutaneous carcinoid tumor

TABLE 3 CLINICAL BEHAVIOR OF MERKEL CELL CARCINOMA

Local recurrence	40%
Average elapsed time before recurrence	10 months
Regional lymph node metastasis	
At presentation	12%
At 12-month follow-up	55%
Distant metastasis (at 9-year follow-up)	36%

From Hitchcock CL, Bland KI, Laney, RG, et al. Neuroendocrine (Merkel cell) carcinoma of the skin: its natural history, diagnosis, and treatment. *Ann Surg* 1988;207:201–207, with permission.

(25%), the lower extremities (18%), and the trunk. Tumors in unusual locations such as the eyelid, lip, and vulva have also been described.

Because of the nonspecific appearance of Merkel cell carcinoma, a broad differential diagnosis exists (Table 2). Merkel cell carcinoma may be clinically confused with basal cell carcinoma, squamous cell carcinoma, amelanotic malignant melanoma, pyogenic granuloma, tumors of adnexal origin, and cutaneous metastases, including breast and lung. Interestingly, Merkel cell carcinoma may coexist with basal cell carcinoma and squamous cell carcinoma in the same anatomic location (Table 3).

Pathogenesis

The pathogenesis of Merkel cell carcinoma has not yet been elucidated. It is likely that ultraviolet light–induced alterations may be causative in the formation of the tumor because over 50% of these tumors are located on the head and neck. With regard to the precise histogenesis of Merkel cell carcinoma, it is unclear whether the tumor arises from epidermal Merkel cells, dermal neuroendocrine cells, or pluripotential epidermal stem cells. The findings of squamous differentiation support an origin from the epidermal stem cell. In contrast, the presence of neurosecretory granules and neuropeptides in Merkel cells supports the likelihood that the tumor is derived from dermal neuroendocrine cells that have migrated from the neural crest.

Diagnosis

To establish the diagnosis of Merkel cell carcinoma, an adequate tissue specimen for standard histopathologic study can be obtained by means of a punch biopsy. Electron microscopy or immunocytochemistry are needed to confirm the diagnosis. Once the diagnosis is established, a complete review of systems and physical examination, including careful palpation of lymph nodes, is essential. A baseline chest radiograph is needed to exclude metastases to the lung. Follow-up studies, including computed tomography scan, are indicated only if there is clinical suspicion of metastases. A careful work-up is mandated because of the aggressive nature of this tumor. At the time of initial diagnosis, 12% of patients have metastases to regional lymph nodes, and metastases develop in another 50% despite treatment.

Histopathology

Light Microscopy

Under light microscopy, Merkel cell carcinoma appears as a dermal nodule with extensions into the underlying subcutaneous fat and muscle. There is usually a clear zone that separates the tumor cells from the epidermis. It consists of a sheet of cells forming nests and cords. The cells are uniform in size with round nuclei and scant cytoplasm. Merkel cell carcinoma has three distinct patterns based on its cellular differentiation (well differentiated, intermediately differentiated, and poorly differentiated). Tumors of the intermediate cell type are the most common. All three types consist of interconnecting trabeculae separated by strands of connective tissue. A high number of mitotic figures are found. There is frequent invasion of lymphatic and vascular spaces by the tumor cells. Areas of squamous differentiation and keratin horn pearls have been described.

Using conventional staining such as hematoxylin and eosin, Merkel cell carcinoma is difficult to distinguish from other tumors such as metastatic oat cell carcinoma of the lung, metastatic carcinoid, cutaneous lymphoma and leukemia, as well as other cutaneous metastases. However, light microscopy is extremely helpful in that if it suggests Merkel cell carcinoma, electron microscopy and immunocytochemistry may then be undertaken to confirm the diagnosis.

Electron Microscopy

Electron microscopy helps to reveal 80- to 100-nm neurosecretory granules peripherally located in the tumor cells. In addition, there are characteristic aggregates of keratin intermediate filaments that are located in a paranuclear fashion. These aggregates are known as "fibrous bodies." The combination of neurosecretory granules and fibrous bodies, in addition to immunocytochemical findings, are important in making the diagnosis of Merkel cell carcinoma.

Immunocytochemistry

Immunocytochemical staining is crucial in establishing the diagnosis of Merkel cell carcinoma. Merkel cell carcinoma has epithelial and neural properties and thus expresses both epithelial and neuroendocrine markers. Neuron-specific enolase is the most consistent marker in Merkel cell carcinoma. Other markers include chromogranin A and synaptophysin, which stain neuroendocrine tumors. Merkel cell tumors may also stain with epithelial membrane antigen and desmoplakin, which serve as evidence for the epithelial differentiation of these tumors.

Another useful marker for the differentiation of Merkel cell carcinoma from other tumors is the keratin monoclonal antibody. A "paranuclear" labeling pattern confirms the diagnosis of Merkel cell carcinoma. A variety of other neuropeptides may be used to detect Merkel cell carcinoma, including chromogranin, synaptophysin, vasoactive intestinal peptide, calcitonin, corticotropin (adrenocorticotropic hormone), met-enkephalin, gastrin, and somatostatin.

In contrast, cutaneous lymphoma should stain with leukocyte common antigen but not with keratin or neuron-specific enolase. Malignant melanoma stains positively with S-100. Although squamous cell carcinoma stains positively for keratin, there is no labeling with neuron-specific enolase. Difficulty in the histologic differentiation of this tumor from oat cell carcinoma of the lung and metastatic carcinoid may be encountered because both of these tumors stain positively for neuron-specific enolase and keratin. However, the diagnosis of Merkel cell carcinoma can be established by the presence of the characteristic paranuclear keratin staining, which is absent in the other tumors.

Treatment

Localized Disease

Because of the aggressive nature of this tumor, an adequate margin of normal tissue is essential to minimize recurrence. The treatment of choice for a localized lesion has been reported to be wide local excision with a 1- to 3-cm margin. Some have advocated the use of Mohs micrographic surgery for management of localized tumor because it allows for microscopically controlled excision of the tumor while sparing normal tissue. Others have argued that because of the high potential for lymphatic and vascular invasion, Mohs micrographic surgery should be reserved only for those tumors located in anatomic areas where sparing of tissue is essential.

Radiation therapy is commonly used as adjunctive treatment after wide local excision of Merkel cell carcinoma. It may also be used for recurrent disease or when there is evidence of angiolymphatic invasion. The radiation field should include the original site of the tumor, the postoperative scar line, and the primary local draining lymph nodes. The use of radiation therapy as the primary modality in the treatment of Merkel cell carcinoma has been advocated for patients who are poor surgical candidates or have large, unresectable tumors located near vital structures.

Regional and Systemic Disease

Local recurrence or regional lymphatic spread carries a very poor prognosis. It has been reported that approximately two thirds of these patients ultimately die of their disease. The treatment of choice in these cases involves excision of the recurrent tumor, lymph node dissection, and radiation therapy of the surgical site as well as the draining lymph nodes. Chemotherapy is the treatment of choice for patients with disseminated Merkel cell carcinoma.

Prognosis

Merkel cell carcinoma is regarded as a highly malignant tumor. The long-term prognosis of these patients is unfavorable (Figs. 2 and 3). Merkel cell carcinoma has a high incidence of local recurrence as well as lymphatic spread. Most local recurrences tend to occur within 1 year of initial diagnosis, with regional lymph node metastases occurring in approximately 50% to 75% of patients. Distant lymphatic spread most frequently involves the liver, bone, brain, lung, and skin (Table

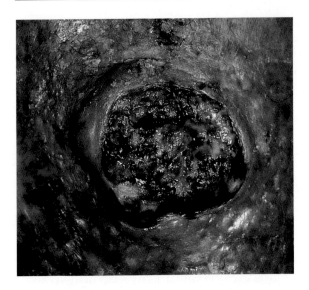

Figure 2

Merkel cell carcinoma: advanced tumor in an immunosuppressed patient. Ulceration and bleeding may be an associated feature.

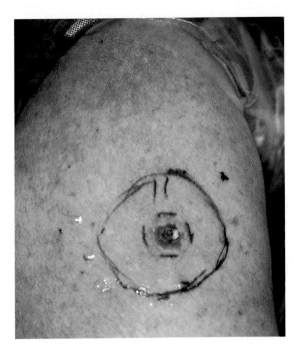

Figure 3

Merkel cell carcinoma. This highly aggressive tumor may mimic multiple other tumors, including squamous cell carcinoma and malignant melanoma.

TABLE 4 COMMON SITES OF DISTANT METASTASIS FOR MERKEL CELL CARCINOMA

Liver
Bone
Brain
Lung
Skin

TABLE 5 SURVIVAL RATES IN PATIENTS WITH MERKEL CELL CARCINOMA

One-year survival	88%
Two-year survival	72%
Three-year survival	55%

4). Unfavorable prognostic factors include tumor larger than 2 cm in diameter, location on the head and neck, histologic evidence of lymphatic and vascular involvement, a poorly differentiated histologic pattern, a mitotic index of 10 per high-power field, and metastases at time of initial diagnosis.

The aggressive nature of this tumor makes close observation even more essential. Patients with Merkel cell carcinoma need meticulous monitoring, with follow-up examinations geared toward the early detection of regional as well as metastatic disease. This may be achieved through a careful review of systems and a skin examination with palpation of lymph nodes, liver, and spleen.

Table 5 lists survival rates in patients with Merkel cell carcinoma.

Suggested Readings

Bayrou O, Avril F, Charpentie P, et al. Primary neuroendocrine carcinoma of the skin. *J Am Acad Dermatol* 1991;24:198–207.

Cotter AM, Gate JO, Gibbs FA. Merkel cell carcinoma: combined surgery and radiation therapy. *Am Surg* 1986;52:159–164.

Goeptert H, Remmler D, Silva E, et al. Merkel cell carcinoma of the head and neck. *Arch Otolaryngol* 1984;110:707–712.

Hanke CW, Conner C, Temofeew RK, et al. Merkel cell carcinoma. *Arch Dermatol* 1989;125:1096–1100.

Hitchcock CL, Bland KI, Laney RG, et al. Neuroendocrine (Merkel cell) carcinoma of the skin: its natural history, diagnosis, and treatment. *Ann Surg* 1988;207:201–207.

Marks ME, Kim RY, Sulter MM. Radiotherapy as an adjunct in the management of Merkel cell carcinoma. *Cancer* 1990;65:60–64.

Meland NB, Jackson IT. Merkel cell tumor: diagnosis, prognosis, and management. *Plast Reconstr Surg* 1986;77:632–638.

Mercer D, Brandler P, Liddell K. Merkel cell carcinoma: the clinical course. *Ann Plast Surg* 1990;25:136–141.

Raaf JH, Urmacher C, Knappa EK, et al. Trabecular (Merkel cell) carcinoma of the skin. *Cancer* 1986;57:178–182.

Roenigk RK, Goltz RW. Merkel cell carcinoma: a problem with microscopically controlled surgery. *Journal of Dermatologic Surgery and Oncology* 1986;12:332–336.

Tennvale J, Biorklund A, Johansson L, et al. Merkel cell carcinoma: management of primary, recurrent and metastatic disease. *Eur J Surg Oncol* 1989;15:1–9.

Wynne CJ, Kearsley JH. Merkel cell tumor: a chemosensitive skin cancer. *Cancer* 1988;62:28–31.

CHAPTER **8**

FIBROHISTIOCYTIC TUMORS

This chapter deals with a group of tumors of mesenchymal origin involving the skin or the superficial soft tissue that are biologically cancerous and exhibit a malignant microscopic morphology. These tumors are extremely rare, especially compared with those cancers that arise from the epidermis, such as basal cell carcinoma and squamous cell carcinoma. Here, we discuss the more common fibrohistiocytic tumors: atypical fibroxanthoma (AFX) and malignant fibrous histiocytoma (MFH).

Atypical Fibroxanthoma

Clinical Features

Atypical fibroxanthoma is an asymptomatic, relatively rare tumor that predominantly arises on the sun-exposed areas in elderly people (Figs. 1 and 2). The head and neck region is most commonly affected, especially the nose and the ears (Fig. 3). Sporadic cases have been reported on the trunk and extremities. AFX usually presents as a small (<2 cm), nonspecific, superficial, solitary red nodule that often ulcerates with time. Because of its occurrence on the sun-damaged skin of the elderly and its nonspecific clinical characteristics, it is commonly mistaken for squamous cell carcinoma or basal cell carcinoma before biopsy (Fig. 4). AFX is generally considered a benign entity, with rare reports of spread to the local draining lymph nodes. Metastasis more commonly occurs in neglected lesions with deep tissue invasion or in immunosuppressed patients.

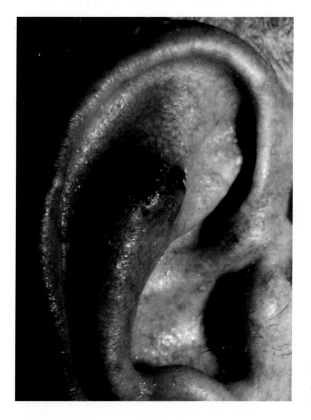

Figure 1
Atypical fibroxanthoma: a small, solitary nodule that often ulcerates with time.

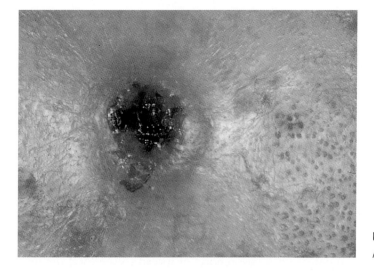

Figure 2
Atypical fibroxanthoma.

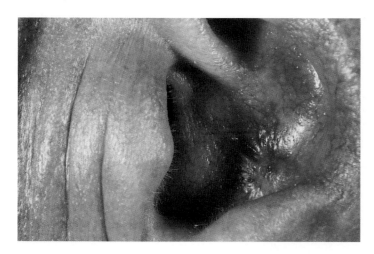

Figure 3
Atypical fibroxanthoma on the ear.

Pathogenesis

The precise pathogenesis of AFX is not known. It is believed that an abnormal proliferation of histiocytes gives rise to this tumor. This is supported by a strong positive reactivity to histiocytic markers. It is generally thought that ultraviolet light plays an essential role in the induction of this tumor based on its occurrence on the sun-damaged skin of elderly people. Irradiation is thought to play a similar role because AFX also occurs in covered areas that have been previously irradiated.

Diagnosis

Because of the location of this tumor on the head and neck and its nonspecific clinical morphology, the differential diagnosis of AFX includes squamous cell car-

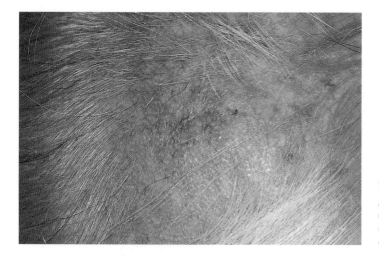

Figure 4
Atypical fibroxanthoma: a flesh-colored papule. This tumor predominantly arises on sun-exposed areas of the elderly.

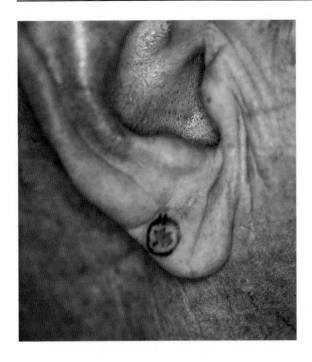

Figure 5

Malignant fibrous histiocytoma: a rare tumor that represents an advanced form of atypical fibroxanthoma. It has a high rate of recurrence, so aggressive intervention is essential.

cinoma, basal cell carcinoma, and amelanotic malignant melanoma. A shave biopsy of this lesion is adequate for histologic diagnosis.

A more difficult problem arises in the differentiation of AFX from MFH (Fig. 5). These two entities may be indistinguishable histopathologically, and many believe that the two entities are closely related. However, the two lesions differ clinically. MFH occurs in younger people, primarily on the extremities and the buttocks. It is a soft tissue tumor that originates in the deep fascia and invades the dermis only secondarily. AFX is generally considered to remain superficial and is thought to be the superficial component of MFH. MFH is considered to be of a much more malignant nature than AFX.

Histopathology

Although not encapsulated, AFX lesions are usually located in the superficial dermis without extension into the underlying subcutaneous fat or fascia. The overlying epidermis is thin with occasional ulceration. A dense cellular infiltrate is present in the superficial dermis. This cell population shows a well-circumscribed

**TABLE 1 HISTOLOGIC DIFFERENTIAL DIAGNOSIS
OF SPINDLE CELL LESIONS OF THE SKIN**

Atypical fibroxanthoma
Squamous cell carcinoma
Malignant melanoma
Malignant fibrous histiocytoma
Dermatofibrosarcoma protuberans

TABLE 2 IMMUNOHISTOCHEMICAL STAINING PATTERNS OF SPINDLE CELL TUMORS OF THE SKIN

	S-100 Protein	Cytokeratins	Vimentin	AAT	AACT
Squamous cell carcinoma	−	+	−	−	−
Malignant melanoma	+	−	+	−	−
Leiomyosarcoma	−	−	+/−	−	−
Malignant fibrous histiocytoma	−	−	−	+	+
Atypical fibroxanthoma	−	−	n/a	+	+

AAT, α_1-antitrypsin; AACT, α_1-antichymotrypsin.

nodular collection of large, bizarre-appearing, multinucleated giant cells with markedly atypical nuclei. Spindle-shaped cells with hyperchromatic nuclei and pleomorphic-appearing histiocytic cells are also present.

Atypical fibroxanthoma lesions may histopathologically resemble and be mistaken for poorly differentiated squamous cell carcinoma or amelanotic malignant melanoma (Table 1). Immunohistochemical staining patterns may aid in their differentiation. The tissue histiocyte markers α_1-antichymotrypsin and α_1-antitrypsin serve to distinguish AFX lesions from these other tumors. Furthermore, there is positive staining for vimentin, a mesenchymal marker. AFX does not express keratin, which is uniformly present in lesions of poorly differentiated squamous cell carcinoma. An absence of S-100 protein staining rules out the diagnosis of malignant melanoma. These immunohistochemical stains are essential to confirm the diagnosis of AFX (Table 2).

Treatment

Surgery is the mainstay of therapy. Conservative excision may be adequate for superficial lesions, but there is a potential for recurrence with the deeper tumors. A recurrence rate of less than 10% has been reported with conservative excision. Tumors that arise in irradiated skin or in immunocompromised patients as well as recurrent tumors should be treated more aggressively. Metastasis is rare, but has been reported. Mohs micrographic surgery with margin control may be advantageous in treating this tumor.

Malignant Fibrous Histiocytoma

Clinical Features

Malignant fibrous histiocytoma is a flesh-colored to red nodule that is rarely diagnosed before excision and histopathologic evaluation. It primarily arises from the skeletal muscle of the extremities or the buttocks in elderly people. MFH is the most common dermal tumor of late adult life.

Histopathology

As alluded to earlier, this tumor may be indistinguishable from AFX histopatho-logically. Spindle cells arranged in a storiform pattern with bizarre giant cells are a common finding. The tumor is poorly demarcated and is situated deep in the dermis.

Pathogenesis

The precise pathogenesis is not established. Studies suggest a mixture of histio-cytic and fibroblast derivation.

Treatment

There is a high rate of local recurrence associated with this tumor, and therefore wide excision has been strongly recommended. Metastasis, especially to the lungs, occurs fairly commonly (>40%), so aggressive intervention on diagnosis is a must.

Suggested Readings

Alguacil-Garcia A, Unni K, Goellner JR, et al. Atypical fibroxanthoma of the skin. *Cancer* 1977;40:1471–1480.

Brown MD, Swanson NA. Treatment of malignant fibrous histiocytoma and atypical fibrous xanthomas with micrographic surgery. *Journal of Dermatologic Surgery and Oncology* 1989;15:1287–1292.

Fretzin DF, Helwig EB. Atypical fibroxanthoma of the skin. *Cancer* 1973;31:1541–1552.

Helwig EB, May D. Atypical fibroxanthoma of the skin with metastasis. *Cancer* 1986;57:368–376.

Jacobs DS, Edwards WD, Ye RC. Metastatic atypical fibroxanthoma of the skin. *Cancer* 1975;35:457–462.

Leong ASY, Milios J. Atypical fibroxanthoma of the skin. *Histopathology* 1987;11:463–475.

Soares HL, Silveira JG, Fantini A, et al. Atypical fibroxanthoma. *Journal of Dermatologic Surgery and Oncology* 1981;7:915–916.

CHAPTER 9

ADNEXAL TUMORS OF THE SKIN

"Adnexa" refers to the appendages of the skin, including eccrine and apocrine sweat glands, sebaceous glands, and hair follicles. Malignancies can and do develop from each of these structures, although they are not very common. They are difficult to identify because of their inconspicuous appearance. Histologic diagnosis may also be somewhat difficult because of their similarity to other benign and malignant skin conditions. This chapter deals with some of the more common adnexal tumors of the skin.

Microcystic Adnexal Carcinoma

Clinical Features

Microcystic adnexal carcinoma (MAC) is a rare tumor of eccrine origin. Although original descriptions found the tumor to occur predominantly in young to middle-aged women, it is now known that the sexes are affected equally and most patients are actually in their sixth and seventh decades. Most cases reported in the literature occur in the upper lip area. The nasolabial folds, the periorbital regions, and the scalp are involved most often. The tumor presents as an inconspicuous, slow-growing, firm, flesh-colored to red nodule. The margins of the tumor are usually difficult to delineate. It is usually asymptomatic, although invasive tumors may cause paresthesia or pain secondary to perineural infiltration.

Microcystic adnexal carcinoma is an aggressive tumor that invades deeply into the subcutaneous tissue and muscle, causing significant destruction. Perineural invasion is frequently observed. Despite the invasive nature of the tumor and its propensity for recurrence, it does not seem to metastasize.

Differential Diagnosis

The clinical features are nonspecific and the differential diagnosis includes morpheaform basal cell carcinoma (BCC), squamous cell carcinoma, acne cyst, and intradermal nevus. A shave biopsy usually is adequate for histologic diagnosis.

Pathogenesis

The origin of this tumor remains uncertain. Many believe the tumor to be of eccrine origin, but others have pointed to a follicular and sweat gland differentiation of the tumor.

Histopathology

The tumor is located in the dermis and often involves the subcutaneous fat. Histologic features include squamous cysts and strands of keratinocytes with ductal differentiation situated in a desmoplastic stroma. Mitoses and cytologic atypia are extremely uncommon. It may histologically resemble morpheaform BCC, where islands of basophilic cells are seen in a fibrous stroma. Doubtful cases may be confirmed by epithelial membrane antigen or carcinoembryonic antigen immunohistochemistry.

Treatment

The mainstay of treatment for sebaceous carcinoma is surgical excision. The indistinct borders and the deeply invasive nature of the tumor contribute to its incomplete removal. Recurrences after excision are common, occurring in over 30% of cases. For this reason, Mohs micrographic surgery with control of tissue margins is highly recommended. Irradiation is not a viable option because it penetrates poorly into the fibrocollagenous tumor stroma, providing inadequate results.

Prognosis

The long-term prognosis for patients with MAC is excellent because of the virtual absence of metastatic spread. Careful follow-up is recommended, however, because of the high rate of recurrence associated with this tumor.

Dermatofibrosarcoma Protuberans

Clinical Features

Dermatofibrosarcoma protuberans (DFSP; Figs. 1–6) is recognized as one of the more common fibrohistiocytic tumors of the skin. Although DFSP more commonly occurs on the trunk of young adults between the third and fifth decades of

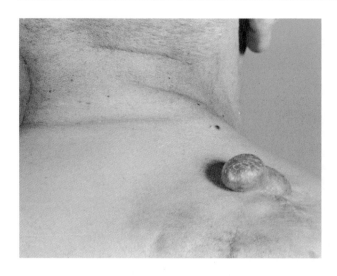

Figure 1

Dermatofibrosarcoma protuberans. A flesh-colored to red multinodular plaque fixed to the overlying skin is characteristic.

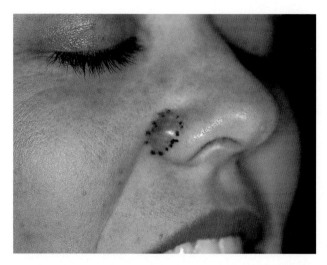

Figure 2

Dermatofibrosarcoma protuberans. Although most common on the trunk, the tumor may be found in all anatomic locations.

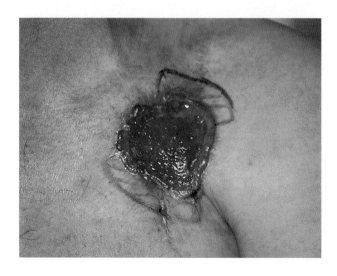

Figure 3

Dermatofibrosarcoma protuberans. This tumor has a tendency toward local recurrence, but reports of metastatic spread are rare.

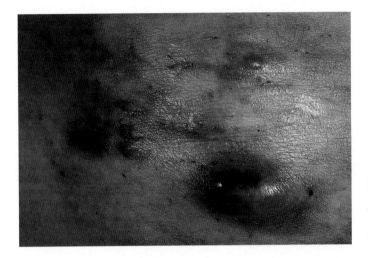

Figure 4

Dermatofibrosarcoma protuberans. The multinodular appearance with a rapid increase in size is characteristic of this tumor.

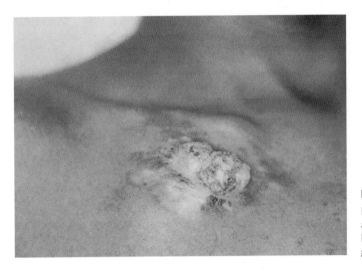

Figure 5

Dermatofibrosarcoma protuberans. This tumor tends to involve beyond the clinically visible margins of the tumor.

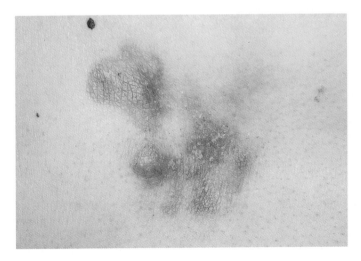

Figure 6

Dermatofibrosarcoma protuberans. This patient was treated with Mohs micrographic surgery, and 5 years later has no evidence of tumor recurrence.

Figure 7
Dermatofibrosarcoma protuberans: an early lesion.

life, it may be found in all anatomic locations and age groups. It usually begins as a flat, violaceous patch that slowly grows into a flesh-colored to red, firm, multinodular plaque that is fixed to the overlying skin (Fig. 7). Tumors may attain a size greater than 20 cm in diameter. Most patients seek medical attention because of a rapid increase in size of the tumor or a new-onset tenderness. There is a greater incidence of this tumor in men. DFSP is considered a low-grade tumor of the skin with a marked tendency for recurrence, but with a very low metastatic potential (Figs. 8–10). Distant metastases have been reported, but are extremely rare.

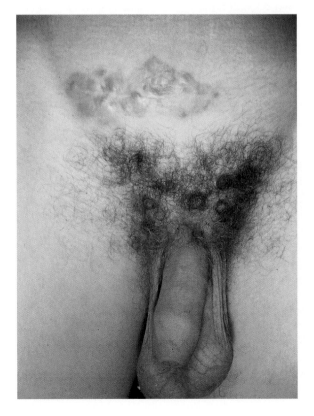

Figure 8
Dermatofibrosarcoma protuberans.

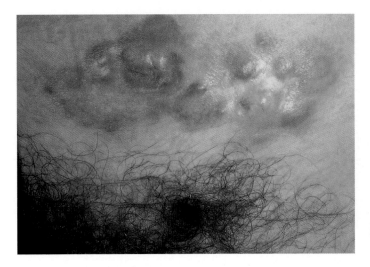

Figure 9
Dermatofibrosarcoma protuberans.

Pathogenesis

The etiology of DFSP remains controversial. Perineural as well as histiocytic origins of this tumor have been described. DFSP has arisen in surgical scars, vaccination sites, and burn scars. Up to 20% of the cases may be preceded by trauma. It remains to be determined whether this association is casual or incidental. Based on electron microscopic findings, the tumor is thought to arise from fibroblasts. Also, DFSP tumor cells have shown considerable type I collagen synthesis in cell culture, which provides further evidence for the fibroblastic origin of this tumor.

Diagnosis

A punch biopsy or incisional biopsy with adequate penetration into the dermis is needed to arrive at a diagnosis.

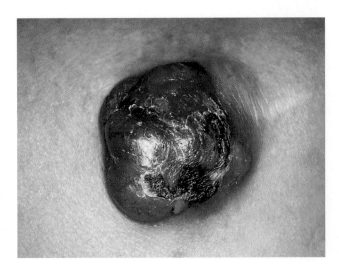

Figure 10
Dermatofibrosarcoma protuberans.

Histopathology

Dermatofibrosarcoma protuberans is predominantly composed of cells with spindle-shaped nuclei packed in a collagen framework of the dermis. These cells are arranged in intertwining bands, resulting in a characteristic storiform pattern. These cells radiate in a whorl-like fashion, which produces a cartwheel-like appearance. A marked degree of cellularity is present, with minimal pleomorphism and mitotic activity. There is usually a zone of normal dermis between the epidermis and the tumor. DFSPs are not encapsulated and often infiltrate deep into the subcutaneous fat, fascia, and underlying muscle, with the tumor spreading along the connective tissue and surrounding the pilosebaceous units. The high recurrence rate of DFSP is due to these peripheral extensions, which have a bland appearance, similar to that of normal collagen. This can make it difficult to determine the exact borders of the tumor. Immunohistochemical markers used to confirm the diagnosis of DFSP include CD34 and vimentin.

Another histologic variant of DFSP is known as the "Bednar tumor." This is the pigmented variant of DFSP and accounts for approximately 5% of all cases reported. Its histologic features are identical to those of DFSP, but with the addition of melanin. Special stains (S-100) may be needed to differentiate this entity from a spindle cell melanoma.

Treatment

Dermatofibrosarcoma protuberans is a locally aggressive neoplasm with a high propensity for recurrence. This is due to the marked involvement of the surrounding dermis and subcutaneous tissue beyond the visible margins of the tumor. A wide surgical excision with at least a 3-cm margin has been the recommended treatment. Despite this, numerous reports of recurrence of the tumor have been documented. Experience with Mohs micrographic surgery has suggested that it may be the treatment of choice for DFSP. Multiple studies have shown the technique to provide high cure rates with maximal preservation of normal tissue.

Desmoplastic Trichoepithelioma

Clinical Features

Desmoplastic trichoepithelioma, also referred to as "sclerosing epithelial hamartoma," is an asymptomatic, solitary, slowly growing, locally invasive tumor. It is usually less than 1 cm in diameter and commonly presents with a raised border and a depressed center. It occurs mainly on the face and neck, especially on the forehead, cheek, and the chin. It most commonly occurs in young men and women, although it has a higher propensity for women.

Pathogenesis

Desmoplastic trichoepithelioma is a hamartomatous tumor of hair follicle origin.

Pathology

Pathologic features include numerous keratin-filled cysts and epithelial strands composed of small, dark tumor cells (one to three cells thick) situated in the upper dermis. A dense fibrous stroma is present between the tumor cells. Mitotic figures are either absent or very rare, and there is no pleomorphism. Focal calcification is a common feature.

Diagnosis

Desmoplastic trichoepithelioma is most commonly confused with morpheaform BCC. There are a number of distinguishing factors because desmoplastic trichoepithelioma lacks the characteristic peripheral palisading and retraction artifact surrounding the tumor cells that is commonly seen in BCC. In addition, BCC lacks the keratin-filled cysts that are commonly found in desmoplastic trichoepithelioma.

Syringoma, a benign entity, and MAC may strikingly resemble desmoplastic trichoepithelioma. A review of the biopsy specimen by an experienced dermatopathologist may be needed to distinguish between these entities.

Treatment

Local excision is effective in most cases. Partial removal is usually followed by regrowth.

Angiosarcoma

Clinical Features

Synonymous with "malignant angioendothelioma" and "lymphangiosarcoma," angiosarcoma is an uncommon, rapidly growing, malignant tumor that is associated with high morbidity and mortality rates (Fig. 11). It may arise from the skin or within the internal organs. The cutaneous form most commonly arises on the face and scalp, with a special predilection for elderly men. It usually presents as a single or multiple purple patches, plaques, or nodules. It has a tendency to ulcerate and bleed. Alternatively, angiosarcoma may rarely arise as a complication of radical mastectomy on a background of chronic lymphedema on the extremities. It may also occur as a late complication of radiation therapy. In these cases, the tumor develops in the vicinity of the zone of radiation and is very aggressive in nature. By the time the diagnosis is made, it has usually penetrated deep into the subcutaneous tissue with metastasis by lymphatic or hematogenous routes. The most common sites of metastasis are the lymph nodes, lungs, and the liver. Clinical presentation is quite variable, as shown in Figures 12 through 15.

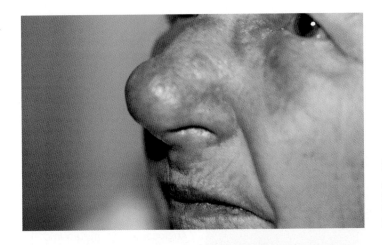

Figure 11

Angiosarcoma: violaceous, rapidly progressive plaque on the face of this elderly man. This is a characteristic presentation.

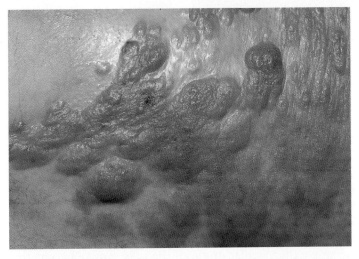

Figure 12

Recurrent angiosarcoma. Recurrence and metastasis of this tumor are very common regardless of the treatment modality.

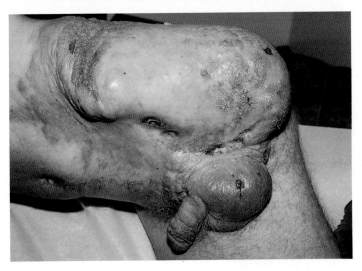

Figure 13

Angiosarcoma: metastatic lesions.

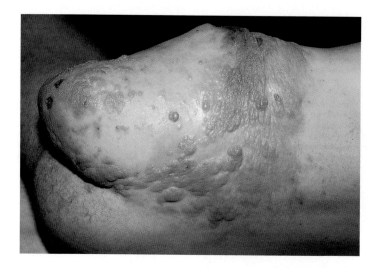

Figure 14
Angiosarcoma: metastatic lesions.

Pathogenesis

Immunohistochemical and ultrastructural analysis have shown this neoplasm to be of endothelial origin.

Histopathology

The histopathologic appearance is variable based on the level of differentiation of the tumor. Dilated, thin-walled, anastomosing vascular channels with plump endothelial cells, nuclear atypia, and frequent mitoses are found infiltrating through the surrounding collagen. The neoplasm often extends deep into the subcutaneous fat and fascia. Staining with monoclonal antibodies to factor VIII–related antigen may be used to prove the vascular origin of the cells. Angiosarcoma that

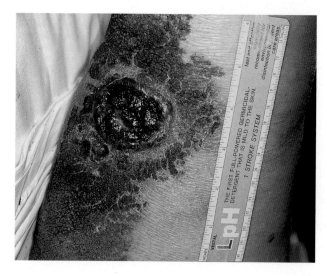

Figure 15
Angiosarcoma.

arises in a background of chronic lymphedema on the extremities does not differ histologically from angiosarcoma of the scalp.

Diagnosis

A biopsy specimen and careful clinicopathologic correlation are needed to confirm the diagnosis of angiosarcoma. Nodular lesions of angiosarcoma may be blue-black in color, and thus may be mistaken for malignant melanoma. Under pathologic examination, careful attention to detail is necessary to avoid mistaking this entity for a benign vascular lesion. Histologically, the tumor may be confused with Kaposi sarcoma and, in some cases, spindle cell melanoma. Once the diagnosis is made, a careful work-up must be undertaken to determine the extent of spread of the tumor.

Treatment

Because of the tumor's tendency to metastasize early in its course, early diagnosis and complete surgical excision are the only hopes for cure. Otherwise, prognosis is poor regardless of the treatment modality. This makes an early diagnosis essential if survival is to be affected. Wide excision and grafting has been helpful in some cases. The response to radiation therapy has been disappointing.

Suggested Readings

Alessi E, Sala F, Berti E. Angiosarcomas in lymphedematous limbs. *Am J Dermatopathol* 1986;8:371–378.

Barnes L, Coleman JA, Johnson JT. Dermatofibrosarcoma protuberans of the head and neck. *Arch Otolaryngol* 1984;110:398.

Bendix-Hansen K, Myhre-Jensen O, Kaae S. Dermatofibrosarcoma protuberans: a clinicopathologic study of nineteen cases and review of world literature. *Scand J Plast Reconstr Surg* 1983;17:247.

Brenner W, Schaefler K, Chhabra H, Postel A. Dermatofibrosarcoma protuberans metastatic to a regional lymph node: report of a case and review. *Cancer* 1975;36:1897–1902.

Brownstein MH, Shapiro L. Desmoplastic trichoepithelioma. *Cancer* 1977;40:2979–2986.

Burkhardt BR, Soule EH, Winkelmann RK, Ivins JC. Dermatofibrosarcoma protuberans: study of 56 cases. *Am J Surg* 1966;111:638–644.

Cooper PH, Mills SE. Microcystic adnexal carcinoma. *J Am Acad Dermatol* 1984;10:908.

Fleischmann HE, Roth RJ, Wood CC, et al. Microcystic adnexal carcinoma treated by microscopically controlled excision. *Journal of Dermatologic Surgery and Oncology* 1984;10:873.

Girard C, Johnson WC, Graham JH. Cutaneous angiosarcoma. *Cancer* 1970;26:868–883.

Goldstein DJ, Barr RJ, Sant Cruz DJ. Microcystic adnexal carcinoma: a distinct clinicopatholgoic entity. *Cancer* 1982;50:566.

Grant RA. Sweat gland carcinoma with metastases. *JAMA* 1960;173:490.

Haltberg BM. Angiosarcomas in chronic lymphedematous extremities. Two cases of Stewart-Treves syndrome. *Am J Dermatopathol* 1987;9:406.

Hashimoto K, Brownstein MH, Jakobiec FA. Dermatofibrosarcoma protuberans: a tumor with perineural and endoneural cell features. *Arch Dermatol* 1974;110:874–875.

Hobbs ER, Wheeland RG, Bailin PL, et al. Treatment of dermatofibrosarcoma protuberans with Mohs micrographic surgery. *Ann Surg* 1988;207:102.

Hodgkinson DJ, Soule EH, Woods JE. Cutaneous angiosarcoma of the head and neck. *Cancer* 1979;44:1106–1113.

Holder CA, et al. Angiosarcoma of the face and scalp, prognosis and treatment. *Cancer* 1987;59:1046.

Lupton GP, McMarlin SL. Microcystic adnexal carcinoma: report of a case with 30-year follow-up. *Arch Dermatol* 1986;122:286.

MacDonald DM, Wilson Jones E, Marks R. Sclerosing epithelial hamartoma. *Clin Exp Dermatol* 1977;2:153.

Maddox JC, Evans HL. Angiosarcomas of the skin and soft tissue: a study of forty-four cases. *Cancer* 1981;48:1907–1921.

Marks LB, Suit HD, Rosenberg AE, et al. Dermatofibrosarcoma protuberans treated with radiation therapy. *Int J Radiat Oncol Biol Phys* 1989;17:379.

McPeak CJ, Cruz T, Nicastri AD. Dermatofibrosarcoma protuberans: an analysis of 86 cases-five with metastasis. *Ann Surg* 1967;166:803–816.

Mehregan AH, Hashimoto K, Rahbari H. Eccrine adenocarcinoma: a clinicopathological study of 35 cases. *Arch Dermatol* 1983;119:104–114.

Mikhail GR, Lynn BH. Dermatofibrosarcoma protuberans. *Journal of Dermatologic Surgery and Oncology* 1978;4:81.

Nickoloff BJ, Fleischmann HE, Carmel J, et al. Microcystic adnexal carcinoma: immunologic observations suggesting dual differentiation. *Arch Dermatol* 1986;122:290.

Robinson JK. Dermatofibrosarcoma protuberans resected by Mohs surgery. *J Am Acad Dermatol* 1985;12:1093.

Taylor HB, Helwig EB. Dermatofibrosarcoma protuberans: study of 115 cases. *Cancer* 1962;15:717.

Weber PJ, Gretzula JC, Hevia O, et al. Dermatofibrosarcoma protuberans. *Journal of Dermatologic Surgery and Oncology* 1988;14:555.

Wick MR, Cooper PH, Swanson PE, Kaye VN, Sunn TT. Microcystic adnexal carcinoma: an immunohistochemical comparison with other cutaneous appendage tumors. *Arch Dermatol* 1990;126:189–194.

CHAPTER 10

TEST SLIDES

Questions

Answers start on page 186.

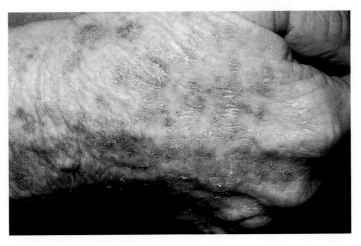

Retired construction worker with keratotic, rough papules on a pink base on the dorsum of the hands.

1a. The most likely diagnosis is?
1b. The most appropriate next step is to?

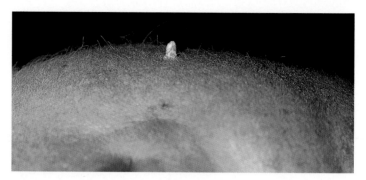

A 42-year-old white man with a "bump" present for 5 months.

2a. The most likely diagnosis is?
2b. The most appropriate next step is to?

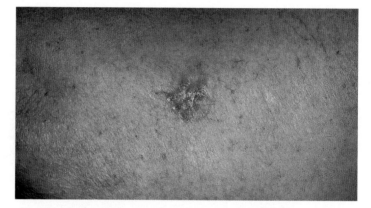

Fair-complected, elderly man with a lesion on the chest that had been slowly developing over a period of years.

3a. The most likely diagnosis is?
3b. The most appropriate next step is to?
3c. What would be the most appropriate treatment modality?

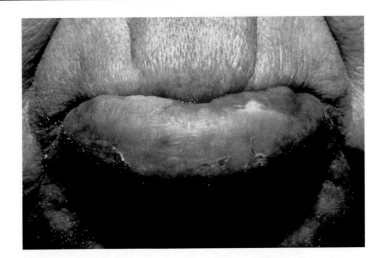

Elderly farmer who gradually noted a white discoloration of his lower lip with occasional crusting

4a. The most likely diagnosis is?
4b. The most appropriate next step is to?

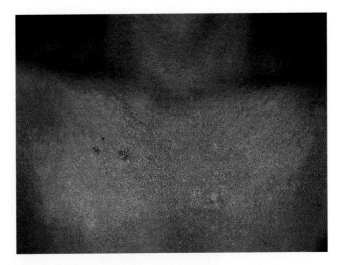

Patient with slowly growing, asymptomatic lesion on the chest.

5a. The most likely diagnosis is?
5b. The most appropriate next step is to?
5c. What would be the most appropriate treatment modality?

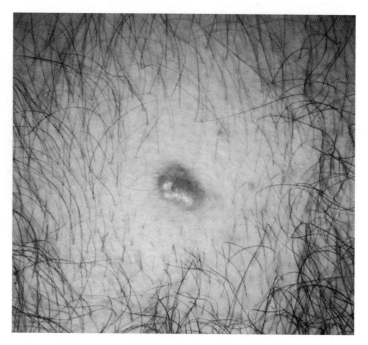

A 73-year-old white man with an asymptomatic papule on the upper back.

6a. The most likely diagnosis is?
6b. The most appropriate next step is to?
6c. What would be the most appropriate treatment modality?

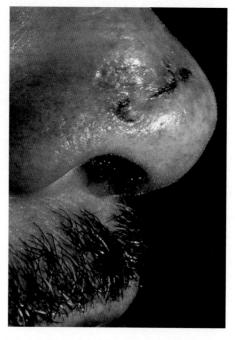

Patient with poorly defined lesion on the right nasal ala.

7a. The most likely diagnosis is?

7b. The most appropriate next step is to?

7c. What would be the most appropriate treatment modality?

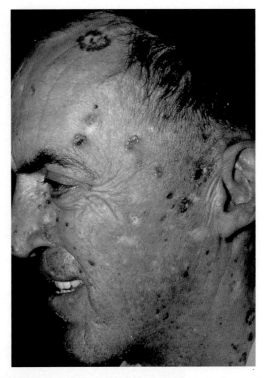

Patient with multiple basal cell carcinomas scattered throughout. He began to have basal cell cancers during his teenage years.

8. Why is the patient developing all of these skin cancers at such an early age?

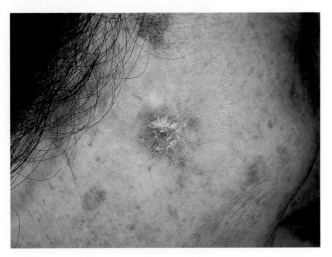

9. Fair-complected, middle-aged woman comes in for evaluation of a persistent lesion present on the right cheek for approximately 2 years.

9a. The most likely diagnosis is?
9b. The most appropriate next step is to?
9c. What would be the most appropriate treatment modality?

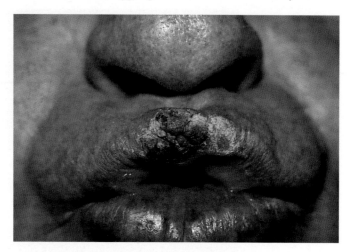

Middle-aged man with crusted nodule on the upper lip.

10a. The most likely diagnosis is?
10b. The most appropriate next step is to?

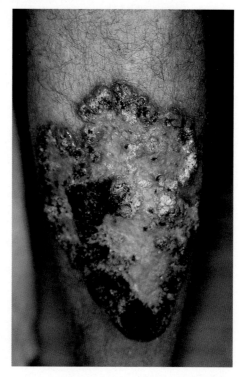

Patient with tumor in a recurrently ulcerated stasis dermatitis of the lower leg present for many years.

11a. The most likely diagnosis is?

11b. The most appropriate next step is to?

11c. What would be the most appropriate treatment modality?

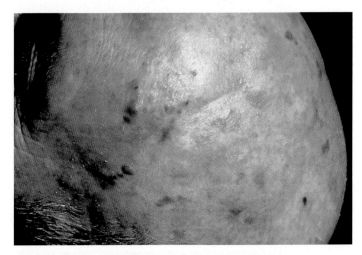

A 63-year-old white man with an erythematous, firm, dome-shaped nodule on the left upper forehead. There are also multiple keratoses.

12a. The most likely diagnosis is?

12b. The most appropriate next step is to?

12c. What would be the most appropriate treatment modality?

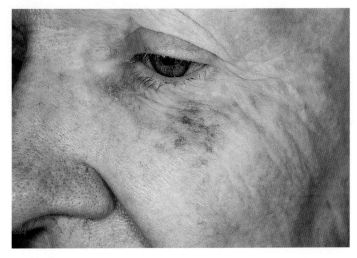

Patient with irregularly pigmented, brown patch on the left infraorbital skin. The lesion had been present for many years.

13a. The most likely diagnosis is?

13b. The most appropriate next step is to?

13c. What would be the most appropriate treatment modality?

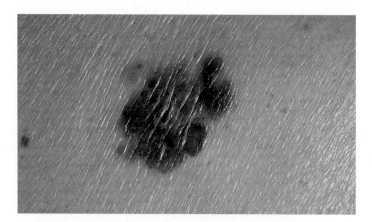

Fair-complected patient with a slowly enlarging lesion on the trunk.

14a. The most likely diagnosis is?
14b. The most appropriate next step is to?
14c. What would be the most appropriate treatment modality?

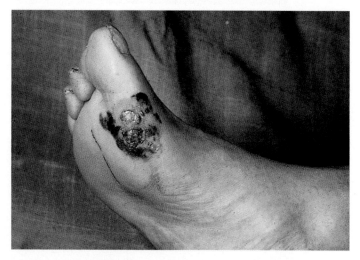

Middle-aged engineer who presented with the complaint of a bruise on his right foot that gradually grew in size.

15a. The most likely diagnosis is?
15b. The most appropriate next step is to?
15c. What would be the most appropriate treatment modality?

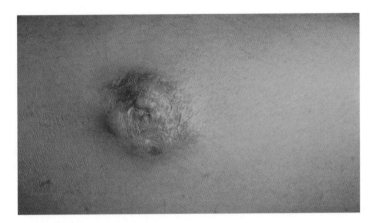

Patient who presented with an asymptomatic, firm nodule.

16a. The most likely diagnosis is?
16b. The most appropriate next step is to?
16c. What would be the most appropriate treatment modality?

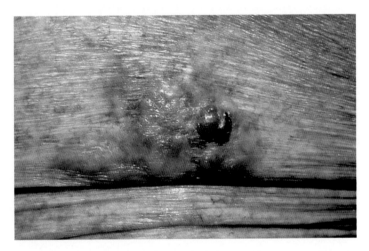

Patient who had been treated with x-ray therapy 40 years earlier, in whom an asymptomatic nodular lesion developed.

17a. The most likely diagnosis is?
17b. The most appropriate next step is to?
17c. What would be the most appropriate treatment modality?

Answers

1a. Actinic keratosis.
1b. Freeze with liquid nitrogen. May consider treatment with topical 5-fluorouracil cream.

2a. Cutaneous horn.
2b. Perform a shave biopsy, making sure to include the base of the specimen. The base of the specimen is needed to make an accurate pathologic diagnosis. In this case, histopathologic evaluation showed an actinic keratosis at the base of the lesion. In other cases, a wart or squamous cell carcinoma may be found at the base of the tumor.

3a. Bowen disease (squamous cell carcinoma-*in-situ*).
3b. Shave biopsy of the specimen confirmed Bowen disease.
3c. Electrodesiccation and curettage or surgical excision would both be appropriate treatment modalities.

4a. Actinic cheilitis.
4b. Freeze the entire lesion with liquid nitrogen. Appropriate follow-up is needed to ensure the lesion does not recur. If resolution is not noted, a biopsy should be considered.

5a. Basal cell carcinoma (superficial).
5b. Perform a shave biopsy of the lesion, which confirms the diagnosis of superficial basal cell carcinoma.
5c. Electrodesiccation and curettage or surgical excision of the tumor are both appropriate treatment modalities.

6a. Basal cell carcinoma (nodular).
6b. Perform a shave biopsy of a portion of the lesion, which confirms the diagnosis of nodular basal cell carcinoma.
6c. Considering the anatomic location of the tumor, referral of patient for Mohs micrographic surgery would be the most appropriate treatment modality.

7a. Sclerosing basal cell carcinoma.
7b. Perform a shave biopsy of the lesion, which confirms the diagnosis of sclerosing basal cell carcinoma.
7c. Because of the aggressive and infiltrative nature of this tumor, the patient should be referred for Mohs micrographic surgery.

8. The patient has the basal cell nevus syndrome. This is an autosomal dominant disorder in which patients develop basal cell carcinomas as early as late childhood. A number of other organs, including bones, soft tissue, eyes, central nervous system, and endocrine organs, may be affected.

9a. Squamous cell carcinoma.
9b. Perform a shave biopsy of the lesion, which confirms the diagnosis of squamous cell carcinoma.
9c. Depending on the size of the tumor, surgical excision or, preferably, Mohs

micrographic excision of the tumor should be considered. For those patients who are poor surgical candidates, radiation therapy may be considered.

10a. Squamous cell carcinoma of the lip.
10b. Perform a shave or punch biopsy of the lesion to confirm clinical suspicion. The biopsy should extend beyond the crust in order for the pathologist to be able to establish a diagnosis.

Squamous cell carcinomas located on the mucosa tend to be more aggressive in nature and at higher risk for spread. An examination of the draining lymph nodes is a mandatory part of the evaluation before proceeding. For lesions that have spread, referral to a head and neck surgeon would be indicated. For lesions confined to the lip, referral for Mohs micrographic surgery is the appropriate next step.

11a. Squamous cell carcinoma (Marjolin ulcer).
11b. Confirm by biopsy.
11c. Squamous cell carcinoma developing in a background of stasis dermatitis tends to be more aggressive than tumors occurring in sun-exposed areas. Aggressive intervention with Mohs micrographic surgery would be indicated.

12a. Merkel cell carcinoma.
12b. Perform a biopsy to confirm clinical suspicion.
12c. Merkel cell carcinoma is a highly malignant tumor with a high incidence of local recurrence as well as lymphatic spread. Wide local excision with a 1- to 3-cm margin of normal tissue has been advocated. For those tumors located in cosmetically sensitive areas, microscopic control with Mohs surgery may be helpful in sparing normal tissue.

13a. Lentigo maligna.
13b. Perform punch biopsy of the darkest, most indurated area of the tumor to establish the diagnosis. Because the biopsy is read as lentigo maligna, the tumor has not yet penetrated beyond the basement membrane and is confined to the epidermis.
13c. The preferred modality of treatment is excision of the entire lesion with margins of normal skin to ensure complete removal. For sundry reasons, including the patient's age, general health, and the cosmetic deformity that may result from a large excision on the face, other treatment modalities have been proposed. These include cryotherapy, laser therapy, and ionizing radiation. All have been associated with higher recurrence rates.

If the tumor had penetrated beyond the basement membrane, excision down to or including the fascia with a 1-cm margin of normal skin would be indicated. For the larger lesions, a skin graft is usually needed for closure of the defect.

14a. Superficial spreading melanoma.
14b. Perform a punch biopsy (incisional biopsy) to establish the diagnosis. (If the lesion is reasonably small and appears suspect, an excisional biopsy—removal of the entire lesion—may be undertaken.)
14c. A full-thickness biopsy and, if at all possible, one that includes the entire lesion, should be submitted for pathologic evaluation. Histopathologic evaluation establishes the thickness of the tumor, which is the primary guideline by which the

surgeon chooses the margin of normal skin that needs to be removed around the tumor. Excisions should always be carried down to the level of the fascia.

15a. Acral lentiginous melanoma.
15b. Perform a punch biopsy to establish the diagnosis (although the clinical presentation is pathognomonic).
15c. In addition to standard surgical excision of the tumor with appropriate margins of normal skin (based on tumor thickness), amputation of the afflicted area, regional lymph node dissection, or regional perfusion with chemotherapeutic agents may be indicated.

16a. Dermatofibrosarcoma protuberans.
16b. Perform a punch biopsy to establish the diagnosis.
16c. Dermatofibrosarcoma protuberans is a locally aggressive neoplasm with a high propensity for recurrence because of its tendency to extend beyond the clinically visible margins of the tumor.

Although a wide surgical excision with 3-cm margins of normal tissue had been advocated in the past, Mohs micrographic surgery appears to be a better therapeutic option.

17a. Angiosarcoma.
17b. Perform a punch biopsy to establish the diagnosis.
17c. This tumor has a tendency to metastasize early in its course. Early diagnosis and wide surgical excision are the only hopes for cure.

Subject Index

Page numbers followed by *t* and *f* indicate tables and figures, respectively.